Immunology of Eye Diseases

IMMUNOLOGY AND MEDICINE SERIES

IMMUNOLOGY

SERIES · SERIES · SERIES · SERIES AND SERIES · SERIES · SERIES · SERIES

MEDICINE

Volume 13

Immunology of Eye Diseases

Edited by
Susan Lightman

Institute of Ophthalmology
University of London
London, UK

Series Editor: Professor Keith Whaley

KLUWER ACADEMIC PUBLISHERS

DORDRECHT/BOSTON/LONDON

Distributors

for the United States and Canada: Kluwer Academic Publishers, PO Box 358, Accord Station, Hingham, MA 02018–0358, USA
for all other countries: Kluwer Academic Publishers Group, Distribution Center, PO Box 322, 3300 AH Dordrecht, The Netherlands

British Library Cataloguing in Publication Data

Immunology of eye diseases.
  1. Man. Eyes. Diseases. Immunological aspects
  I. Lightman, Susan II. Series
  617.7′1

IBSN 0–7923–8908–5

Copyright

Published in the United Kingdom by Kluwer Academic Pubishers, PO Box 55, Lancaster, UK.

Kluwer Academic Publishers BV incorporates the publishing programmes of D. Reidel, Martinus Nijhoff, Dr W. Junk and MTP Press.

Printed in Great Britain by Butler & Tanner Ltd, Frome and London.

This book is dedicated to Professor Sir Stanley Peart for his enthusiasm, commitment and support for the subject of ocular immunology.

It has been a great privilege to work with so many people with different specialist interests while putting this book together. I have learned a great deal in the process and I hope that it will stimulate both ophthalmologists and scientists to think further about these problems, which present major management problems in our clinical practice.

Susan Lightman,
London, February 1989

Contents

List of Contributors

D. A. BREWERTON
Department of Rheumatology
Charing Cross and
Westminster Medical School
17 Page Street
London SW1P 2AP
UK

R. R. CASPI
Laboratory of Immunology
National Eye Institute
National Institutes of Health
Bethesda
Maryland 20892
USA

CHI-CHAO CHAN
Laboratory of Immunology
National Eye Institute
National Institutes of Health
Bethesda
Maryland 20892
USA

C. CLAOUÉ
Department of Ophthalmology
St Thomas' Hospital
London SE1 7EH
UK

K. FAIRBURN
Department of Rheumatology
Bloomsbury Rheumatology Unit
Middlesex Hospital
Arthur Stanley House
Tottenham Street
London W1P 9PG
UK

M. G. FALCON
St Thomas' Hospital
London SE1 7EH
UK

D. A. FRANCIS
Department of Neurology
Guy's Hospital
St Thomas' Street
London SE1 9RT
UK

A. GARNER
Department of Pathology
Institute of Ophthalmology
17/25 Cayton Street
London EC1V 9AT
UK

S. HOWIE
University of Edinburgh
Department of Pathology
University Medical School
Teviot Place
Edinburgh EH8 9AG
UK

D. I. ISENBERG
Department of Rheumatology
Bloomsbury Rheumatology Unit
Middlesex Hospital
Arthur Stanley House
Tottenham Street
London W1P 9PG
UK

S. LIGHTMAN
Institute of Ophthalmology
17/25 Cayton Street
London EC1V 9AT
UK

A. McCARTNEY
Department of Pathology
Institute of Ophthalmology
17/25 Cayton Street
London EC1V 9AT
UK

W. I. McDONALD
Institute of Neurology
The National Hospital
Queen Square
London WC1N 3BG
UK

Preface

The eye can become involved in immune-mediated diseases that affect it alone or as part of a multi-organ disease process. Much immunological attention has been focused on other organs affected by these processes and the subject of the immunology of eye diseases is a relatively new one. Many of these diseases that involve the eye are not life-threatening but can result in devastating loss of sight that if bilateral, will have major effects on the patient's life. Systemic immunological investigations are generally unhelpful in these patients and one of the major problems in this field has been the lack of diseased tissue available for examination to determine the pathological processes involved.

Our poor understanding of basic mechanisms of disease in the eye has meant that treatment of many of these conditions is often inadequate. It has become possible to apply in the eye many of the techniques used to investigate the role of the immune system in other systems. Animal models of many of the disease processes have also allowed dissection of the immune response both within and outside the eye. It is my belief that a greater understanding of the mechanisms by which the structures in the eye become damaged will allow more specific and effective therapeutic strategies to be devised.

This book aims to cover some of the areas in which there have been significant advances in our knowledge of pathogenesis, based on fact rather than on hypothesis. It does not set out to cover everything and the clinical information is summarized rather than being a main component of each chapter. Discussion of treatment is included only when it is based on the new information. Aspects of the whole spectrum of immune-mediated eye conditions are covered, from corneal grafting to autoimmunity to systemic diseases affecting the eye and the optic nerve. The chapters are written by both clinicians and scientists, in some cases together, with expertise in their respective fields and it has been their choice as to the exact direction of their contributions.

1
Immunogenetics of Eye Diseases

D. A. BREWERTON

In many respects, the problems of ophthalmologists and rheumatologists are similar. A central enigma in both specialties is a group of inflammatory disorders that behave as if they result from infection but in which no living microorganisms have been found. For most of this century, causative organisms have been sought in the eyes and the joints with only limited success. As a result, many theories have been proposed to explain conditions such as acute anterior uveitis and rheumatoid arthritis.

The key to understanding acute anterior uveitis came with the discovery in 1973 that individuals with the inherited transplantation antigen HLA B27 are approximately 20 times as likely as other people to develop this acute inflammatory disorder[1,2]. The association was shown to be particularly strong in the uveitis of Reiter's disease, and so it was assumed that there was probably a subtle defect in handling certain microorganisms or their remnants. At approximately the same time, it was found that people with B27 are also 50–100 times as likely to develop ankylosing spondylitis or the arthritis of Reiter's disease[3-7].

Since then, worldwide population studies have shown that the gene and the uveitis (or arthritis) are about equally associated in virtually all races and populations. This and other evidence indicates that B27 must be directly involved in the disease process.

The fact that an inherited molecule, B27, which is present in 7% of a Caucasian population, is so strongly associated with certain inflammatory disorders in the eyes and joints suggests that acute anterior uveitis is an excellent model for understanding many other diseases.

ANTIGEN RECOGNITION

There are two main systems in the body that recognize and respond to foreign or abnormal materials: the immunoglobulins (antibodies) expressed by B lymphocytes, and the receptors expressed by T lymphocytes, which recognize foreign peptides bound to HLA molecules in antigen-presenting cells.

Crystallographic studies of antigen–antibody complexes have shown that small foreign molecules are bound in clefts in antibody molecules. These clefts are lined by amino acids of variable segments of the immunoglobulin light and heavy chains. Larger antigens are bound to flat surfaces of the antibody molecules.

HLA molecules, which are related to acute anterior uveitis, are not involved in antigen-antibody complexes but in the controlled degradation, selection and presentation of foreign antigens within antigen-presenting cells[8-11]. Most antigens are unable to stimulate T lymphocytes unless they are first processed by antigen-presenting cells (including macrophages, bone-marrow-derived dendritic cells and vascular endothelial cells), which may increase by 1000-fold the ability of antigens to activate T lymphocytes and thereby initiate an inflammatory response (Figure 1.1). The antigen is first endocytosed, and then markedly altered so that the form that stimulates lymphocytes is unlike the original antigen. The antigen is then degraded in a process that ceases when the antigen fragments reach the size of hepta- or octapeptides, otherwise there would be nothing left to stimulate the lymphocytes. It is at this stage that the peptides are bound to the HLA molecules in the antigen-presenting cells and the peptide to be presented is selected (Figure 1.2).

HLA MOLECULES

Recent crystallographic studies[12] have established the detailed three-dimensional structure of HLA molecules (Figure 1.3a and b). Surprisingly, an HLA molecule has a single binding site, a complicated groove in which a substance has been identified as a foreign peptide. Any suitable foreign peptide is non-covalently bound to the groove by complementary conformations. Because there are relatively few different HLA molecules and an almost infinite number of foreign antigens, each type of HLA molecule, such as B27, must be capable of binding several thousand different foreign peptides.

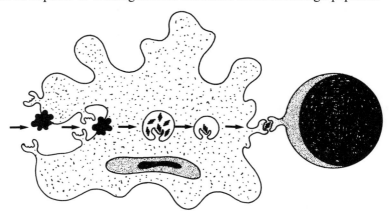

Figure 1.1 A foreign antigen is recognized by an antigen-processing cell. The antigen is edocytosed, degraded, selected, bound to HLA molecules, and presented to a T lymphocyte

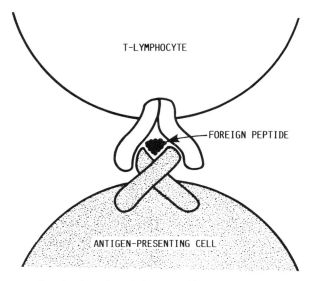

T-LYMPHOCYTE

FOREIGN PEPTIDE

ANTIGEN-PRESENTING CELL

Figure 1.2 After an antigen has been degraded to a peptide and bound to an HLA molecule, it is presented to a T lymphocyte. There is then interaction between the HLA molecule, the T lymphocyte-receptor molecule and the foreign peptide

T LYMPHOCYTE RECEPTOR MOLECULES

In 1974, it was established that T lymphocytes respond to foreign antigens only when the antigen is presented in association with HLA molecules[13]. There is now believed to be an inherent affinity between T lymphocyte receptor molecules and HLA molecules, probably resulting from development together early in their evolution. In consequence, a T lymphocyte can recognize simultaneously whether an antigen-presenting cell is self and whether the peptides bound in its HLA molecules are foreign[11]. The receptors on cyotoxic T lymphocytes recognize Class I HLA molecules, while helper T lymphocytes recognize Class II HLA molecules. Once stimulated, the lymphocytes determine the exquisite specificity of the inflammatory response.

HEREDITY

Superficially, the genetics of HLA, T lymphocyte-receptor and immunoglobulin molecules resembles that of ABO blood groups, but it is immensely more complicated and highly polymorphic. All three members of this genetic superfamily have repertoires of millions of combinations, which together help to characterize us as individuals. The genes for HLA molecules are on the 6th chromosome; the genes for T lymphocyte receptor molecules are on the 2nd, 7th and 14th chromosomes; and the genes for immunoglobulin molecules are on the 2nd, 14th and 22nd chromosomes.

(a)

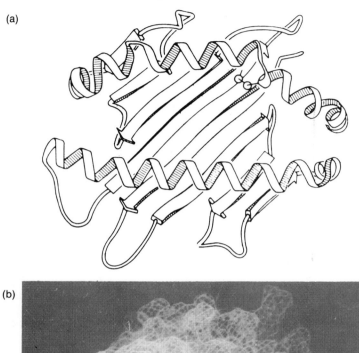

(b)

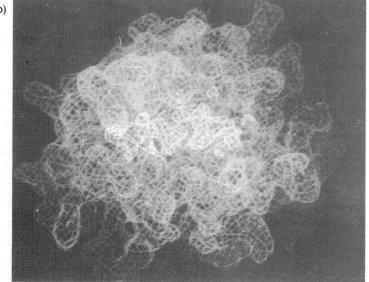

Figure 1.3 (a) Schematic presentation of the structure of an HLA molecule. **(b)** The deep grove identified as the recognition site of an HLA molecule. The light area in the centre represents a bound molecule, probably a peptide. (Reprinted by permission from *Nature*, Vol. 329, pp. 506–12. Copyright © 1987 Macmillan Magazines Ltd.)

For historical and technical reasons, identification of HLA molecules in individuals has been studied intensively as part of tissue-typing. As a result, the associations between HLA molecules and susceptibility to disease have

4

been investigated in patients, in countries, and in races throughout the world. By comparison, similar identification of T lymphocyte-receptor and immunoglobulin polymorphisms is still in its infancy[14].

HLA DISEASE ASSOCIATION

Since the discovery of the association between HLA B27 and diseases of the joints and eyes, various HLA molecules have been found to be associated with a long list of diseases as diverse as multiple sclerosis and psoriasis, haemachromatosis and narcolepsy, coeliac disease and diabetes mellitus, pemphigus and Sjögren's syndrome, myasthenia gravis and thyrotoxicosis, erythema nodosum and Behçet's disease[15].

In most of these associations, the mechanism leading to disease remains totally obscure.

ASSOCIATIONS WITH EYE DISEASES

Of the diseases listed above, multiple sclerosis, diabetes mellitus, Sjögren's syndrome, myasthenia gravis, thyrotoxicosis and Behçet's disease have obvious implications for ophthalmology.

Acute anterior uveitis and its association with HLA B27 remains the only example of a strong association with a disease that is often confined to the eye. The initial report has been confirmed in several studies[16-19].

HLA associations with optic uveitis, ocular histoplasmosis, Birdshot retinochoroidopathy[20], recurrent corneal herpes and the iridocyclitis of juvenile chronic arthritis are widely accepted, while the apparent associations with Vogt–Koyanagi–Harada syndrome, Thygeson's superficial punctate keratitis and hereditary optic atrophy require confirmation[15].

Failures to find associations have been reported in primary open-angle glaucoma, acute angle-closure glaucoma, capsular glaucoma, pigmentary glaucoma, pigment dispersion syndrome, Eales' disease, stromal dystrophy, Fuch's endothelial dystrophy, keratoconus, Cogan's syndrome, scleritis, toxoplasmic retinochoroiditis, retinitis centralis serosa, chorioretinitis, senile cataract, steroid-induced cataract, degenerative choroidopathy, retinitis pigmentosa, rhegmatogenous retinal detachment, sympathetic ophthalmia, pseudoexfoliation of the lens capsule, and Adie's syndrome[16].

In ocular tissues, Class I HLA molecules are expressed in the vascular endothelium. Opinions differ as to whether other ocular tissues express Class I or Class II HLA molecules in the absence of disease[21,22].

ACUTE ANTERIOR UVEITIS

Attempts have been made to establish the clinical features and prognosis of acute anterior uveitis in people with B27 compared with those who do not have B27[2,15,23-25]. Those with B27 have a more severe unilateral anterior uveitis, frequently associated with fibrin in the anterior chamber and the absence of mutton fat keratic precipitates. The inflammation usually persists for 6 weeks and often recurs after long intervals, with a high incidence of ocular complications. The age of onset is often between 20 and 30 years, and is younger than in people without B27.

With an onset of acute anterior uveitis below the age of 40 years. approximately 45% of the men and 25% of the women have clinical evidence of ankylosing spondylitis. In the men under 40 years who have B27, this figure increases to 75%.

Clinically, this type of uveitis is also associated with peripheral arthritis, psoriasis, ulcerative colitis and Crohn's disease.

Despite the strong association between acute anterior uveitis and B27, there is evidence that only 1% of the population with B27 develop eye disease. By contrast, approximately 20–30% of people with B27 and ankylosing spondylitis have acute anterior uveitis at some time. This strongly suggests an additional factor linked to ankylosing spondylitis that has not yet been identified. In a recent family study[26], the frequency of acute interior uveitis in B27-positive individuals was 13% in relatives of patients with acute anterior uveitis and 1% in those with no family history of uveitis, indicating that the missing factor is probably genetic. Similarly, ankylosing spondylitis occurs in only 1% of the B27 population, but in over 20% of the B27 first-degree relatives of probands with ankylosing spondylitis, suggesting a missing genetic component linked to B27.

Interestingly, when acute anterior uveitis is associated clinically with ankylosing spondylitis or peripheral arthritis, the frequency of B27 approaches 100%. By contrast, when ankylosing spondylitis (or acute anterior uveitis) is clinically associated with psoriasis, ulcerative colitis or Crohn's disease, the frequency of B27 falls to 65%, suggesting that the genes for skin and bowel disease can substitute for B27 in inducing susceptibility to joint or eye disease.

The implication of the clinical evidence is that the basic process in acute anterior uveitis is more complicated than the involvement of HLA B27 molecules within antigen-presenting cells. One proposal is that other genes and chromosomes may be involved, and that there may be sophisticated variations in the other members of the genetic superfamily — the T lymphocyte receptors and immunoglobulins[14].

ACUTE ANTERIOR UVEITIS AS A DISEASE MODEL

Since the discovery of the association between acute anterior uveitis and B27, this disorder has been of considerable interest to both rheumatologists and immunogeneticists.

One advantage of studying uveitis, rather than arthritis, is that there is usually a clear-cut onset. Very approximately, half are otherwise fit and half have rheumatic disease, while half have B27 and half do not. This is ideal for conducting epidemiological investigations. Several studies have shown uveitis following epidemics of dysentery with known bacteria such as *Yersinia enterocolitica*. In another survey[27], a persistent T lymphopenia developed in

6

patients, and a transient T lymphopenia was identified in asymptomatic household contacts, suggesting lateral transmission of a viral infection.

The central role of HLA molecules within antigen-presenting cells raises several possibilities in the pathogenesis of uveitis. The marked alteration of foreign substances and their degradation to short peptide chains could explain why microorganisms have not been identified. And the fact that an HLA molecule, such as B27, can bind several thousand different foreign peptides implies that large numbers of diverse antigens might lead to the same clinical response in different individuals or at different times in the same individual.

After an attack of uveitis in one eye, the next few attacks may be in the same one before there is an attack in the opposite eye. By analogy with experimental arthritis, one explanation of this clinical observation could be that there is persistent damage to small blood vessels, possibly facilitating the passage of antigen-presenting cells into the uveal tract.

THE FUTURE

There is certain to be rapid progress in understanding the three-dimensional crystallographic structure of HLA molecules and the mechanisms by which HLA molecules bind with foreign peptides and interact with T lymphocyte receptors. In time, certain T lymphocyte receptors may prove to be critical in regulating precise clinical and immune responses.

References

1. Brewerton, D. A., Caffrey, M., Nicholls, A. *et al.* (1973). Acute anterior uveitis and HL-A27. *Lancet*, **2**, 994–6
2. Brewerton, D. A. (1975). HL-A27 and acute anterior uveitis. *Ann. Rheum. Dis.* **34** (Suppl. 1), 33–5
3. Brewerton, D. A., Caffrey, M., Hart, F. D. *et al.* (1973). Ankylosing spondylitis and HL-A27. *Lancet*, **1**, 904–7
4. Schlosstein, L., Terasaki, P. I., Bluestone, R. *et al.* (1973). High association of an HL-A antigen, W27, with ankylosing spondylitis. *N. Engl. J. Med.*, **228**, 704–6
5. Brewerton, D. A., Caffrey, M., Nicholls, A., Walters, D., Oates, J. K., and James, D. C. O. (1973). Reiter's disease and HLA-27. *Lancet*, **2**, 996–8
6. Brewerton, D. A., Caffrey, M., Nicholls, A. *et al.* (1974). HL-A27 and the arthropathies associated with ulcerative colitis and psoriasis. *Lancet*, **1**, 956–8
7. Brewerton, D. A. (1976). HLA-B27 and the inheritiance of susceptibility to rheumatic disease. *Arthritis Rheum.*, **19**, 656–68
8. Page, R. C., Davies, P. and Allison, A. C. (1974). Participation of mononuclear phagocytes in chronic inflammatory diseases. *J. Reticuloendothelial Soc.*, **15**, 413–38
9. Werdelin, O. (1986). Determinant protection. A hypothesis for the activity of immune response genes in the processing and presentation of antigens by macrophages. *Scand. J. Immunol.*, **24**, 625–36
10. Unanue, E. R. and Allen, P. M. (1987). The basis for the immunoregulatory role of macrophages and other accessory cells. *Science*, **236**, 551–7
11. Marrack, P. and Kappler, J. (1987). The T-cell receptor. *Science*, **238**, 1073–9
12. Bjorkman, P. T., Saper, M. A., Samraoui, B., Bennett, W. S., Strominger, J. L. and Wiley, D. C. (1987). Structure of the human class I histocompatibility antigen, HLA-A2. *Nature*, **329**, 506–12
13. Zinkernagel, R. M. and Doherty, P. C. (1974). Restriction of in vitro T-cell mediated

cytotoxicity in lymphocytic choriomeningitis within a syngeneic or allogeneic system. *Nature,* **248**, 701–2

14. Brewerton, D. A. (1984). A reappraisal of rheumatic diseases and immunogenetics. *Lancet,* **2**, 799–802
15. Tiwari, J. L. and Terasaki, P. I. (1985). *HLA and Disease Associations.* (New York: Springer-Verlag)
16. Mapstone, R. and Woodrow, J. C. (1975). HL-A27 and acute anterior uveitis. *Br. J. Ophthalmol.,* **59**, 270–5
17. Scharf, J., Miller, B., Scharf, J. *et al.* (1976). HL-A27 antigen associated with uveitis and ankylosing spondylitis in a family. *Am. J. Ophthalmol.* **82**, 139–40
18. Saari, M., Miettinen, R., Tiilikainen, A. *et al.* (1977). Acute anterior uveitis and HLA-B27 in families. *Can. J. Ophthalmol.,* **12**, 4–11
19. Beckingsdale, A. B., Davies, J., Gibson, J. M. and Rosenthal, A. R. (1984). Acute anterior uveitis, ankylosing spondylitis, back pain and HLA-B27. *Br. J. Ophthalmol.,* **68**, 741–5
20. Priem, H. A., Kijlstra, A., Noens, L., Baarsma, G. S., De Lacy, J. J. and Oosterhuis, J. A. (1988). HLA typing in Birdshot chorioretinopathy. *Am. J. Ophthalmol.,* **105**, 182–5
21. Bakker, M. and Kijlstra, A. (1985). Expression of HLA-antigens in the human anterior uvea. *Curr. Eye Res.,* **4**, 599–604.
22. Abi-Hanna, D., Wakefield, D. and Watkins, S. (1988). HLA antigens in ocular tissues. *Transplantation,* **45**, 610–13
23. Miettinen, R. and Saari, M. (1977). Clinical characteristics of familial acute anterior uveitis. *Can. J. Ophthalmol.,* **12**, 1–3
24. Linssen, A. (1987). Acute anterior uveitis, ankylosing spondylitis and HLA-B27. Thesis. (The Hague, Opmeer Offset BV)
25. Rothova, A., van Veenendaal, W. G., Linssen, A. *et al.* (1987). Clinical features of acute anterior uveitis. *Am. J. Ophthalmol.,* **103**, 137–45
26. Derhaag, P. J. F. M., Linssen, A., Broekema, N., de Waal, L. P. and Feltkamp, T. E. W. (1988). A familial study of the inheritance of HLA-B27-positive acute anterior uveitis. *Am. J. Ophthalmol.,* **105**, 603–6
27. Byrom, N. A., Campbell, M. A., Hobbs, J. R. *et al.* (1979). T and B lymphocytes in patients with acute anterior uveitis and ankylosing spondylitis, and in their household contacts. *Lancet,* **2**, 601–3

2
Bullous Disorders of Skin Affecting the Conjunctiva

S. LIGHTMAN

INTRODUCTION

Many of the acquired blistering disorders of the skin, which are thought to have an immune basis, also involve the mucous membranes, which include the conjunctiva. In some of these disorders, conjunctival disease may occur asymptomatically and extensive scarring can occur before the patient is aware of any damage. Inflammation in the conjunctiva can lead to loss of goblet cells and poor mucin secretion, scarring of the lacrimal ductules, with reduced tear secretion and cicatricial entropion. The tear film becomes unstable and inadequate, resulting in drying of the cornea, and further damage to the cornea occurs as a result of the inwardly directed lashes. These changes are progressive and are often accompanied by secondary infection. The cornea becomes scarred and vascularized and perforation followed by endophthalmitis may occur.

All of these disorders have specific immunopathological features that are used in diagnosis. The target area for the immune processes is the basement membrane zone of the epidermal–dermal junction and the intercellular substance, which seem to be highly antigenic. The initiating events are not known, but antibodies are formed to different parts of this region that have damaging effects either directly or by complement fixation when interaction occurs with the target antigen. The clinical features of disease are determined by the systemic distribution of the target antigen and the exact site of damage within this zone. For further understanding of the basement membrane zone, the reader is referred to Figure 2.1, which is a simplified drawing of the structures within the dermal–epidermal junction.

CICATRICIAL PEMPHIGOID

Cicatricial pemphigoid is characterized by erosive, scarring, subepidermal blistering lesions of the mucous membranes, particularly of the eye and

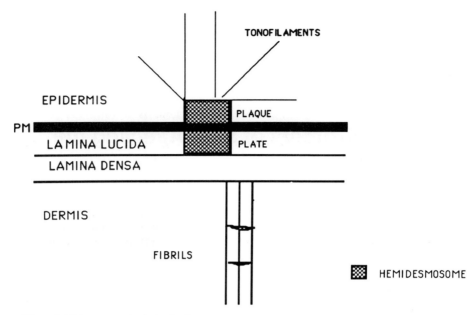

Figure 2.1 Diagram to show detail of basement membrane zone of dermal–epidermal junction of skin. PM = plasma membrane

mouth. Conjunctival scarring occurs in at least 70% of patients with this disorder and may lead to total blindness. Blisters are rarely seen in the eye, but surface ulceration results in progressive fibrosis beneath the conjunctival epithelium and symblepharon formation[1]. This is associated with a diminished tear film since the progressive fibrosis occludes the lacrimal and accessory gland ducts, leading to decreased aqueous tear formation. In addition, the conjunctival scarring results in destruction of the mucin-producing goblet cells and mucin deficiency, which causes instability of the tear film. Entropion, trichiasis and abnormal blinking add to the corneal problems and keratinization of the corneal and conjunctival epithelia eventually occur[2].

In the early stages of the disease, granulation tissue is present under the conjunctival epithelium, with a cellular infiltrate composed mainly of lymphocytes, plasma cells, occasional eosinophils but relatively few neutrophils. Later, there is marked fibrosis with a mononuclear cell component[3,4]. It is seen by electron microscopy that blister formation occurs at the lamina lucida between the plasma membranes of the basal cells and the electron-dense basal lamina. Linear immunoglobulin deposition on the conjunctival basement membrane in the region of the lamina lucida is a characteristic feature of cicatricial pemphigoid, although it is only present in 20–67% of patients[5-7] and deposition of a variety of complement components (C3, C1q, C4, properdin) has also been described[7]. Immunoglobulin deposition in the conjunctiva is seen in other conditions, such as Mooren's

10

ulcer and staphylococcal keratitis, but the deposits are said to be granular rather than linear[7].

Although antibody can be detected bound to the affected basement membrane, circulating autoantibody is not detected in most patients with cicatricial pemphigoid when using standard substrates[8], but when fresh conjunctiva was used, such antibodies were found in some of the patients[9]. Passive transfer of disease to animals by serum from affected individuals does not occur. It has been suggested that pemphigoid is attributable to an insoluble antigen attached to the basement membrane of the epithelium (which is localized by electron microscopy to the region of the lamina lucida, below that of the bullous pemphigoid antigen)[10] and that an antibody-mediated complement dependent reaction produces cytotoxic reactions (type II) at the tissue site[11].

Elevated levels of immune complexes were found to occur in 31% of blister fluids although only 17% of the sera of these patients had circulating immune complexes. Anti-basement membrane zone antibody was found in 57% of the precipitated complexes from the blister fluids, perhaps suggesting that the majority of the immune complexes are formed *in situ*[12].

Immunoglobulins and complement are also bound to the conjunctival epithelium in cicatricial pemphigoid[11], which suggests that an antigen-antibody reaction is taking place. Circulating antibodies that bind to the conjunctival and corneal epithelium but not to the basement membrane have also been described[7]. Autoantibodies of both the IgG and IgA type have been described in pemphigoid[13]. With the IgG antibodies, fixation to the basement membrane may be followed by the binding of complement to that site. Neutrophils can then be attracted into the site and further damage occurs. The desmosomal attachments of the basal layers of the epithelium to the basement membrane appear to be lysed by an immunological process that results in cellular destruction. It is not known whether these autoimmune phenomena are involved in the pathogenesis of this disease or whether they are formed as a consequence of the tissue destruction.

Patients with cicatricial pemphigoid have an increased frequency of HLA-B12[14], although this association has been questioned in a recent study (P. Wright, personal communication). A decrease in the number of circulating T cells has been reported in patients with cicatricial pemphigoid[15], but the non-specific suppressor functions of the patients' suppressor T cells appears to be intact[16].

PEMPHIGUS VULGARIS

Pemphigus vulgaris is an intra-epidermal blistering disorder which, although it occurs in all races, is particularly common in the Jewish race. The blisters are very fragile and break easily leaving areas of denuded skin that generally heal without scarring. Any area of skin may be involved and more than 90% of patients develop oral lesions[17]. Immunofluorescent studies have shown marked regional variations in expression of pemphigus vulgaris antigen and it is thought that the clinical distribution of lesions in pemphigus vulgaris

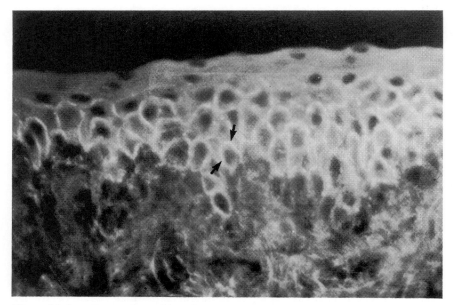

Figure 2.2 *Pemphigus vulgaris*. Direct immunofluorescence of perilesional skin demonstrating inter-epidermal cell deposits of C3 (arrows). Frozen section × 280 (Courtesy of Mr G. Haffenden)

reflects this. All stratified squamous epithelial mucosal sufaces may become involved, including the conjunctiva. Peripheral blood eosinophilia has been reported to occur in 45% of patients[18].

Eighty to ninety per cent of patients with pemphigus have circulating IgG antibodies directed against the intercellular cement substance, as identified by indirect immunofluorescence. All four subclasses of IgG have been observed[19]. The titre of circulating antibody has been found by some groups to correlate with the degree of disease activity[20] but not by others[21]. It is suggested that this difference may be due to the different sensitivities of the substrate used for the detection of the antibodies and the frequency with which the samples are taken[22]. Linear IgG deposits are found in the intercellular space on biopsied perilesional skin by direct immunofluorescence. Thirty to fifty per cent of patients have IgM or IgA deposition and up to 50% have C3 deposition in the intercellular space (Figure 2.2). The immune deposits are most intense in deep acantholytic areas[21].

The pemphigus vulgaris antigen has been the subject of much work and sera from these patients were shown to react with a 210 kDa antigen isolated and characterized from cultured human epidermal cells[23]. The precise nature of the antigen *in vivo* still remains a mystery.

This is an intra-epithelial disorder in which the primary event is thought to be dissolution of the intercellular cement substance with dissolution of the desmosomes occurring as a secondary event[24]. Electron microscopy indicates that the earliest discernible pathological event is the dissolution of the desmosomes. As it is intra-epithelial, scarring and adhesions of the conjunctiva occur only rarely and the main association is with a purulent conjunctivitis[25]. However, shearing of the skin on the eyelids may occur as a result of manoeuvring the lid to insert antibiotic drops (P. Wright, personal communication). Immunofluorescence studies have shown intercellular deposition of IgG in the conjunctival epithelium[25] and circulating antibodies that bind to the intercellular space of the epidermis are found in the sera of almost all patients with pemphigus[26].

Pemphigus may occur during therapy with penicillamine. It is not clear whether the drug is providing carrier help through direct modification of the autoantigen or of some independent molecule concerned in associative recognition. In most cases, the eruption has resolved on cessation of the drug[27].

Both *in vivo* and *in vitro* studies support the pathogenetic role of pemphigus antibodies in the induction of acantholysis[17]. Pemphigus occurs in neonates born to mothers with the disease, but there is spontaneous resolution of the disease by several weeks of age when the maternal antibody titres are decreasing. The IgG fraction of pemphigus serum can induce acantholysis in cultured human keratinocytes. Whole IgG fractions of pemphigus serum injected into neonatal mice were able to induce blistering and erosions with histopathological and immunofluorescent features identical to human disease. Antibodies to purified human pemphigus vulgaris antigen were raised in rabbits and when given IP to normal rabbits were able to induce disease identical to that seen in man. Some of these antibodies have been shown to fix complement and Sams and Schur[28] showed that the pemphigus antibody activity resides in the subclasses of IgG that fix complement. In other studies, complement was not necessary for the pathological effect of the antibody but was thought to augment the pathogenicity of the pemphigus autoantibodies under certain conditions[29]. Low total haemolytic complement and individual complement components have been found in pemphigus blister fluids[30]. Circulating immune complexes have been detected, as has an elevated serum C1q binding activity, but are thought to be a consequence of rather than the cause of the tissue damage[31]. Other cell types including eosinophils (especially in early lesions), neutrophils and T lymphocytes may also infiltrate the tissue and augment the acantholysis[32].

The plasminogen activator urokinase has been demonstrated in perilesional skin in pemphigus vulgaris. It is suggested that the keratinocytes that have been damaged by the autoantibody release urokinase themselves and that this results in the acantholysis by breaking down the intercellular cement substance[33].

BULLOUS PEMPHIGOID

Bullous pemphigoid classically affects older people (although it can rarely occur in children) and is characterized by tense blisters that may rupture, leaving eroded areas that do not tend to spread as occurs in pemphigus[34]. The distribution of skin lesions is influenced by regional variations in the bullous pemphigoid antigen[35]. Mucous membrane involvement may occur and may be

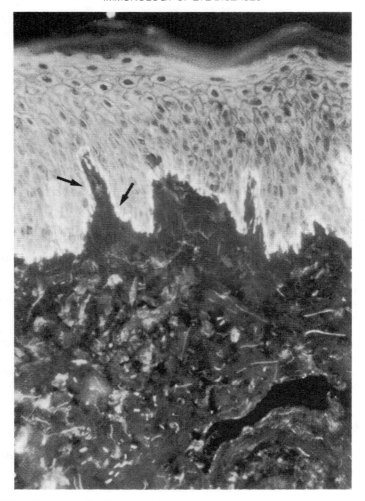

Figure 2.3 *Bullous pemphigoid.* Direct immunofluorescence of perilesional skin showing linear band of IgG along basement membrane (arrows). Frozen section × 160 (Courtesy of Mr G. Haffenden)

asymptomatic in the conjunctiva, with conjunctival scarring and symblepharon formation[36]. There are no HLA or systemic associations. Peripheral blood eosinophilia and raised IgE are found in about 50% of patients[37].

IgG (Figure 2.3) and C3 are deposited in a linear fashion at the epidermal basement membrane zone in perilesional skin. Subtyping shows that IgG_4 subclass is found in most patients followed by IgG_1 and IgG_3 subclasses. IgA and IgM may also be found and rarely IgE and IgD[38]. About 70% of patients have circulating IgG antibodies to the basement membrane zone, but there is no correlation between the antibody titre and clinical state[39]. Immunoelectron microsopy reveals deposition in the upper portion of the lamina lucida. The bullous pemphigoid antigen is found extracellularly in the lamina lucida and intracellularly in association with the hemidesmosomes[40]. It has been partially characterized as a 200 kDa protein that is thought to be produced by the basal cells and deposited in the basement membrane zone[41]. Antibody alone, in the absence of other inflammatory mediators, does not result in bullous pemphigoid blister formation, in sharp contrast to the situation in pemphigus[42]. In one study, bullous pemphigoid IgE was injected into rabbit corneas. Binding of antibody and complement to the basement membrane zone was demonstrated and neutrophils were seen in the same region[43].

Many complement components, including C3 (most frequent), C1q, C4, C5 and the membrane attack complex of C5-9, have been observed at the basement membrane zone, at times in the absence of immunoglobulin. In addition, blister fluids have been found to contain reduced levels of total haemolytic complement as well as reduced levels of each component[44]. Circulating immune complexes can be detected, but current opinion is that they are secondary to tissue injury[45].

Increased serum and blister fluid IgE levels have been reported. Mast cells can be found adjacent to the basement membrane zone in bullous pemphigoid lesions and elevated levels of histamine and the mast cell enzymes arginine esterase and a Hageman factor cleaver, may be detected in the blister fluid. Eosinophils may also accumulate and degranulate, releasing several proteolytic enzymes. *In vitro* data suggest that dermoepidermal junction separation in bullous pemphigoid can be blocked by proteinase inhibitors. Lymphocytes are also found in this region and lymphokines with chemotractant activity and lymphotoxin-like activity have been detected in the blister fluids[37].

ERYTHEMA MULTIFORME

Erythema multiforme is an acute erythematous inflammatory disorder that can be confined to the skin or more commonly involves the mucosal surfaces as well. A wide variety of precipitating factors have been described—infection with herpes simplex, *Mycoplasma pneumoniae*, reactions to drugs such as sulphonamides, barbiturates, salicylates and phenytoin, and malignancy to name some of them, although in some cases no precipitating factor has been identified. Although all mucous membranes may be involved, the mouth and the eyes are the most severely affected[46].

The acute phase of ocular involvement lasts about 2 weeks with swelling, ulceration and crusting of the lids. The conjunctival involvement varies from mild, which terminates without sequelae, to severe with membrane and pseudomembrane formation and subsequent healing with symblepharon formation. The classic lesion of erythema multiforme is the target lesion in which the central area of the lesion is normal. In the conjunctiva, similar-looking lesions may occur, except that the centre part of the lesion is necrotic. Conjunctival scarring may result in entropion with trichiasis and reduced tear secretion from lacrimal and accessory lacrimal gland duct obstruction and

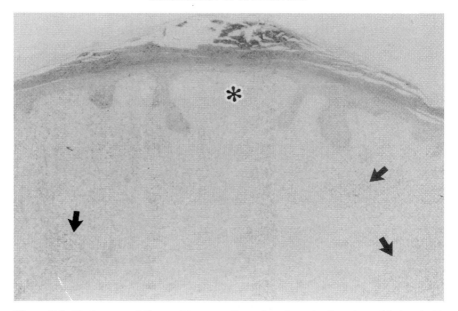

Figure 2.4. *Erythema multiforme.* Haematoxylin and eosin stained section of lesional skin showing perivascular infiltration with mononuclear cells (arrows). Marked oedema resulting in subepidermal blisters (star). × 28 (Courtesy of Mr G. Haffenden)

from goblet cell destruction[47]. Progressive scarring does *not* occur in this condition as it does with cicatricial pemphigoid[2].

In affected conjunctiva as in the skin, there is perivascular infiltration with lymphocytes (Figure 2.4), and pseudomembranes may form that consist of fibrinous exudate, inflammatory cells and necrotic epithelial cells. True membranes result from severe necrotizing reactions when there is sloughing of the conjunctival epithelium and subepithelial layers[47]. In the skin (in the dermal type of disease) and other mucosal areas such as the tracheal mucosa, widespread necrosis of arterioles and venules with fibrinoid degeneration of associated collagen has been described, suggesting that this may be a hypersensitivity reaction. Skin biopsies of erythema multiforme lesions occasionally show deposition of IgM, C3 and fibrin in the superficial vasculature. In addition, immune complexes, both circulating in the blood and in blister fluid, have been detected in a large proportion of these patients[48]. One study suggested that herpes simplex antigens might be part of the complexes[49], but this has never been confirmed. Another study demonstrated that erythema multiforme serum supported herpes simplex-specific cellular cytotoxicity reactions and it is possible that cells containing the virus could become targets for antibody-dependent cellular cytotoxic mechanisms resulting in the lesions of erythema multiforme[50].

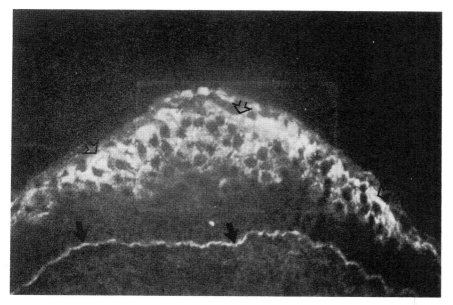

Figure 2.5 *Linear IgA disease*. Bulbar conjunctival biopsy of a patient with cicatrizing conjunctivitis. Direct immunofluorescent staining shows IgA being normally secreted in the mucin (arrowheads) and abnormally deposited along the basement membrane (arrows). Frozen section × 280 (Courtesy of Mr G. Haffenden)

LINEAR IgA DISEASE

Linear IgA disease is characterized by a rash with spontaneous blistering and the presence, in uninvolved areas of skin, of homogeneous linear deposits of IgA along the dermal–epidermal junction (Figure 2.5). There is a high incidence of mucous membrane lesions and in one study over 50% of the patients had changes of cicatrizing conjunctivitis that were often asymptomatic and were clinically indistinguishable from cicatricial pemphigoid[51].

Features of the disorder also overlap with dermatitis herpetiformis. Granular deposition of IgA, particularly in the dermal papillae, is characteristic of dermatitis herpetiformis, in which there is a higher incidence of both an associated enteropathy and HLA B8—over 80% of patients with dermatitis herpetiformis are HLA B8+ as compared to 56% of patients with linear IgA disease[52]. Linear IgA disease has been considered by some to be a subgroup of bullous pemphigoid, with IgA as opposed to IgG being deposited in uninvolved skin. The incidence of circulating anti-basement membrane zone antibodies in the sera of patients with linear IgA disease is low in contrast to bullous pemphigoid. There was, however, a high incidence of other autoantibodies directed at other non-organ-specific targets, suggesting a possible autoimmune basis for the disorder[53].

About 30% of the patients had circulating immune complexes containing IgA, although it is likely that most of the immune complexes are formed locally. Using immunoelectron microscopy, two different sites of IgA deposition can be seen in patients with homogeneous linear deposits, suggesting two subgroups, but the clinical significance of this is unclear. The IgA deposits in skin in dermatitis herpetiformis (DH) contain J chain and are able *in vitro* to bind secretory component. This implies that the IgA is dimeric and likely to have arisen from a mucosal surface, probably the gut. Ninety per cent of the IgA in the serum is in the monomeric form that is produced by non-mucosal sites. IgM also has J chain as it circulates as a pentamer. In most patients with linear IgA disease, there was no J chain present in the IgA deposits, suggesting that the IgA in patients with linear IgA disease is qualitatively different from that of patients with DH[52]. Further evidence of this difference is found on genetic analysis. In linear IgA disease, 53% of patients had HLA-DR3 antigen as compared with 26% of controls, whereas this antigen was present in 88% of patients with DH. Restriction fragment-length polymorphism data focus attention on the DQ region, with DQα 6.2 kb and 6.8 kb fragments in patients with linear IgA disease being very different from that found in controls and in patients with dermatitis herpetiformis[54].

EPIDERMOLYSIS BULLOSA

Epidermolysis bullosa, which can be inherited or acquired, has a wide clinical spectrum and may mimic any of the diseases described above. Mucous membrane involvement is uncommon but can occur. In the eye, cicatrizing conjunctival changes can occur that are often localized and tend not to be progressive[2].

Immunoglobulin (particularly IgG but IgA and IgM have been found) and complement components (C3, C1q, C4) are found at the basement membrane zone by direct immunofluorescence, both in the skin and in mucous membranes. The immune deposits within the basement membrane zone in this disorder are below the lamina densa zone, in contrast to those in bullous pemphigoid, which are above the lamina densa in the lamina lucida region[55]. The antigen in epidermolysis bullosa is a 290 kDa glycoprotein that has been shown to be type VII procollagen. This has a globular carbohydrate domain in the lamina densa and a collagen tail that extends into the sub-lamina densa space, and these tails are thought to be anchoring fibrils[56]. In this disorder, the number of anchoring fibrils as seen by electron microscopy of lesional skin, is greatly reduced.

Circulating anti-basement zone antibodies are detectable in 25–50% of patients, but passive transfer of the disease in animals has not been achieved. *In vitro* evidence suggested that these autoantibodies can fix complement and induce neutrophil migration, which implies that these antibodies do play a role in the pathogenesis of this disorder[57].

Acknowledgements

I would like to thank Mr Peter Wright, Dr Jonathan Leonard and Mr Gerald Haffenden for their invaluable help in putting this chapter together.

References

1. Hardy, K., Perry, H., Pingree, G. and Kirby, T. (1971). Benign mucous membrane pemphigus. *Arch. Dermatol.* **104**, 467–75
2. Wright, P. (1986). Cicatrizing conjunctivitis. *Trans. Ophthalmol. Soc. U.K.* **105**, 1–17
3. Norn, M. S. and Kristensen, E. B. (1974). Benign mucous membrane pemphigoid. II. Cytology. *Acta Ophthalmol.* **52**, 282–90
4. Andersen, S., Jensen, O., Kristensen, E. and Norn, M. (1974). Benign mucous membrane pemphigoid. III. Biopsy. *Acta Ophthalmol.* **52**, 455–63
5. Bean, S. F., Furey, N., West, C. E., Andrews, T. and Esterly, N. B. (1976). Ocular cicatricial pemphigoid. *Trans. Am. Acad. Ophthalmol. Otolaryngol.* **81**, 806–14
6. Furey, N., West, C. E., Andrews, T., Paul, P. D. and Bean, S. F. (1975). Immunofluorescent studies of ocular cicatricial pemphigoid. *Am. J. Ophthalmol.* **80**, 825–31
7. Mondino, B. J., Brown, S. I. and Rabin, B. S. (1978). Autoimmune phenomena of the external eye. *Ophthalmology* **85**, 801–17
8. Rogers, R., Perry, H., Bean, S. and Jordan, H. (1977). Immunopathology of cicatricial pemphigoid. *J. Invest. Dermatol.* **68**, 39–43
9. Leonard, J., Hobday, C., Haffenden, G., Griffiths, C., Powles, A., Wright, P. and Fry, L. (1988). Immunofluorescent studies in ocular cicatricial pemphigoid. *Br. J. Dermatol.* **118**, 209–17
10. Fine, J., Neises, G. and Katz, S. (1984). Immunofluorescence and immunoelectron microscopic studies in cicatricial pemphigoid. *J. Invest. Dermatol.* **82**, 39–43
11. Griffiths, M., Fukuyama, K., Tuffanelli, D. and Silverman, S. (1974). Immunofluorescent studies in mucous membrane pemphigoid. *Arch. Dermatol.* **109**, 195–9
12. Ahmed, A., Moy, R., Chia, D. and Barnett, E. (1983). Immune complexes in pemphigus and bullous pemphigoid. *Dermatologica* **166**, 175–80
13 Sams, W. and Logan, W. (1973). The skin as reflector of immunologic diseases. In Ehrlich, G. (ed.): *Oculocutaneous Manifestations of Rheumatic Diseases*, p. 98. (Basel: Karger)
14. Mondino, B. J., Brown, S. I. and Rabin, B. S. (1979). HLA antigens in ocular cicatricial pemphigoid. *Arch. Ophthalmol.* **97**, 479–83
15. Mondino, B., Rao, H. and Brown, S. (1981). T and B lymphocytes in ocular cicatricial pemphigoid. *Am. J. Ophthalmol.* **92**, 536–42
16. King, A., Schwartz, S., Lopatin, D., Voorhees, J. and Diaz, L. (1982). Suppressor cell function is preserved in pemphigus and pemphigoid. *J. Invest. Dermatol.* **79**, 183–5
17. Korman, C. (1988). Pemphigus. *J. Am. Acad. Dermatol.* **18** (6), 1219–38
18. Crotty, C., Pittelkow, M. and Muller, S. (1983). Eosinophilic spongiosis. *J. Am. Acad. Dermatol.* **8**, 337–43
19. Moy, R. and Jordan, R. (1983). Immunopathology in pemphigus. *Clin. Dermatol.* **1**, 72–82
20. Fitzpatrick, R. and Newcomber, V. (1980). The correlation of disease activity and antibody titres in pemphigus. *Arch. Dermatol.* **116**, 285–90
21. Judd, K. and Lever, W. (1979). Correlation of antibodies in skin and serum with disease severity in pemphigus. *Arch. Dermatol.* **115**, 428–32
22. Beutner, E. (1987). Correlation of pemphigus antibody titres and severity of disease. In Beutner, E., Chorzelski, T. and Kumar, V. (eds.) *Immunopathology of the Skin*, 3rd Edn. (New York: Wiley)
23. Stanley, J., Koulu, L. and Thivolet, C. (1984). Distinction between pemphigus antigens binding pemphigus vulgaris and pemphigus foliaceus autoantibodies. *J. Clin. Invest.* **74**, 313–20
24. Lever, W. F. and Shaumburg-Lever, G. (1975). *Histopathology of the Skin*, pp. 108–17. (Philadephia: Lippincott)
25. Bean, S. F., Holubar, K. and Gillett, R. B. (1975). Pemphigus involving the eyes. *Arch. Dermatol.* **111**, 1484–6
26. Beutner, E. and Jordan, R. (1964). Demonstration of skin antibodies in sera of pemphigus vulgaris patients by indirect immunofluorescent staining. *Proc. Soc. Exp. Biol. Med.* **117**, 505–10
27. Kaplan, R. and Callen, J. (1983). Pemphigus associated diseases and induced pemphigus. *Clin. Dermatol.* **1**, 42–71
28. Sams, W. and Schur, P. (1973). Studies of the antibodies in pemphigoid and pemphigus. *J. Lab. Clin. Med.* **82**, 249–54

19

29. Anhalt, G., Till, G., Diaz, L., Labib, R., Patel, H. and Eaglstein, N. (1986). Defining the role of complement in experimental pemphigus vulgaris in mice. *J. Immunol.* **137**, 2835–40
30. Jordan, R., Day, N., Luckasen, J. and Good, R. (1973). Complement activation in pemphigus vulgaris blister fluid. *Clin. Exp. Immunol.* **15**, 53–63
31. Lawley, T. and Hall, R. (1981). Circulating immune complexes in dermatologic disease. *Springer Seminars in Immunopathology* **4**, 221–40
32. Iwatsuki, K., Tagami, H. and Yamada, M. (1983). Pemphigus antibodies mediate the development of an inflammatory change in the epidermis. *Acta Dermatol. Venereol. (Stockholm)* **63**, 495–500
33. Hashimoto, K., Shafran, K., Webber, P., Lazarus, G. and Singer, K. (1983). Anti-cell surface pemphigus autoantibody stimulates plasminogen activator activity of human epidermal cells. *J. Exp. Med.* **157**, 259–72
34. Lever, W. (1965). Pemphigus and pemphigoid. *J. Am. Med. Assoc.* **200**, 751–6
35. Goldberg, D., Sabolinski, M. and Bystryn, J. (1984). Regional variations in the expression of bullous pemphigoid antigen and location of lesions in bullous pemphigoid. *J. Invest. Dermatol.* **82**, 326–8
36. Venning, V., Frith, P., Bron, A., Millard, P. and Wojnarowska, F. (1988). Mucosal involvement in bullous and cicatricial pemphigoid. *Br. J. Dermatol.* **118**, 7–15
37. Korman, N. (1987). Bullous pemphigoid. *J. Am. Acad. Dermatol.* **16**, 907–24
38. Ahmed, R., Maize, J. and Provost, T. (1977). Bullous pemphigoid. *Arch. Dermatol.* **113**, 1043–6
39. Sams, W. and Jordan, R. (1971). Correlation of pemphigoid and pemphigus antibody titres and activity of disease. *Br. J. Dermatol.* **84**, 7–13
40. Regnier, M., Vaigot, P., Michel, S. and Prunieras, M. (1985). Location of bullous pemphigoid antigen in isolated human keratinocytes. *J. Invest. Dermatol.* **85**, 187–90
41. Stanley, J., Woodley, D. and Katz, S. (1984). Identification and partial characterisation of pemphigoid antigen extracted from normal human skin. *J. Invest. Dermatol.* **82**, 108–11
42. Pehamberger, H., Gshnait, F., Konrad, K. and Holubar, K. (1980). Bullous pemphigoid, herpes gestationes and linear dermatitis herpetiformis. *J. Invest. Dermatol.* **74**, 105–8
43. Anhalt, G., Bahn, C., Labib, R., Voorhees, J., Sugar, A. and Diaz, L. (1981). Pathogenetic effects of bullous pemphigoid autoantibodies on rabbit corneal epithelium. *J. Clin. Invest.* **68**, 1097–101
44. Dahl, M., Falk, R., Carpenter, R. and Micheal, A. (1984). Deposition of the membrane attack complex of complement in bullous pemphigoid. *J. Invest. Dermatol.* **82**, 132–5
45. Yancey, K. and Lawley, T. (1984). Circulating immune complexes: their immunochemistry, biology and detection in selected dermatologic and systemic diseases. *J. Am. Acad. Dermatol.* **10**, 711–31
46. Tonnenson, M. and Soter, N. (1979). Erythema multiforme. *J. Am. Acad. Dermatol.* **1**, 357–64
47. Howard, G. M. (1963). The Stevens–Johnson syndrome: Ocular prognosis and treatment. *Am. J. Ophthalmol.* **55**, 893–900
48. Bushkell, L., Mackel, S. and Jordon, R. (1980). Erythema multiforme: Direct immunofluorescence studies and detection of circulating immune complexes. *J. Invest. Dermatol.* **74**, 372–4
49. Kazmierowski, J. and Wuepper, K. (1982). Herpes simplex antigen in immune complexes of patients with erythema multiforme. *J. Am. Med. Assoc.* **247**, 2547–50
50. Fritz, K., Norris, D., Ryan, S., Huff, J. and Weston, W. (1982). Herpes specific cellular cytotoxicity induced by erythema multiforme serum. *J. Invest. Dermatol.* **78**, 343–4
51. Leonard, J., Wright, P., Williams, D., Gilkes, J., Haffenden, G., McMan, R. and Fry, L. (1984). The relationship between linear IgA disease and benign mucous membrane pemphigoid. *Br. J. Dermatol.* **110**, 307–14
52. Mobacken, H., Kastrup, W., Ljungall, K., Lofberg, H., Nilsson, L., Svensson, A. and Tjernlund, H. (1983). Linear IgA dermatosis. *Acta Dermatol. Venereol. (Stockholm)* **63**, 123–8
53. Leonard, J., Haffenden, G. and Ring, N. (1987). Linear IgA dermatosis in adults. In: Beutner, E., Chorzelski, T. and Kumar, V. (eds.) *Immunopathology of the Skin* 3rd Edn. (New York: Wiley)
54. Sachs, J., Leonard, J., Awad, J., McClosky, D., Festenstein, H., Hitman, G. and Fry, L. (1988). A comparative serological and molecular study of linear IgA disease and dermatitis

herpetiformis. *Br. J. Dermatol.* **118**, 759–64

55. Holubar, K., Wolff, K., Konrad, K. and Beutner, E. (1975). Ultrastructural localization of in vivo bound immunoglobulins in bullous pemphigoid. *J. Invest. Dermatol.* **64**, 47–9

56. Woodley, D., Briggaman, R., O'Keefe, E., Inman, A., Queen, L. and Gammon, W. (1984). Identification of the skin basement autoantigen in epidermolysis acquisita. *N. Engl. J. Med.* **310**, 1007–13

57. Woodley, D. (1988). Epidermolysis bullosa acquisita. *Prog. Dermatol.* **22**, 1–13

3
Immunological Aspects of Anterior Segment Disease of the Eye Induced by Herpes Simplex Virus

C. CLAOUÉ and S. HOWIE

It is perhaps slightly depressing to consider that a submicroscopic virus that has been extensively investigated and whose structure is known to the extent that its entire genome has now been sequenced is still capable of causing devastation to a human eye. Since humans depend on their visual system for some 80% of their total sensory input, damage to the eye is disproportionately severe in relation to similar pathology elsewhere. Unfortunately, although we know a great deal about both the herpes simplex virus and the human eye, our understanding of the interactions that occur when one meets the other are considerably more restricted, and these limitations are reflected by the sadly all too common therapeutic failures.

HERPES SIMPLEX VIRUS

There are six known human herpes viruses including the two serotypes of the alpha herpes virus, herpes simplex. Herpes simplex virus (HSV) normally causes a relatively brief localized primary infection of the epidermis that may pass unnoticed. The virus is of particular importance as a pathogen because during primary infection it travels up axons and establishes latency within neuronal cell bodies of the ganglion innervating the infected dermatome. Once established in the ganglion, the virus may remain latent during the individual's lifetime, or it may periodically reactivate, travel back down axons and cause asymptomatic virus shedding (recurrence) or actual disease (recrudescence) at the peripheral site (reviewed in ref. 1). HSV infections of the immunocompromised (including neonates, genetically or therapeutically immunosuppressed individuals, AIDS patients and certain atopic individuals) can be disseminated rather than localized, and may be life-threatening, illustrating the importance of a competent host immune response in controlling the infection under normal circumstances (reviewed in ref. 2).

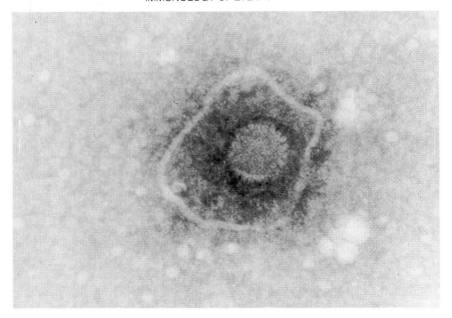

Figure 3.1 Electron micrograph of herpes simplex virion, showing envelope surrounding icosahedral nucleocapsid. Original magnification, × 250 000

STRUCTURE OF HSV

The two serotypes of HSV (HSV-1 and HSV-2) are antigenically related and have approximately 47% genomic homology. The virus has an icosahedral capsid of 100 nm diameter that encloses the double-stranded linear DNA genome. The capsid is surrounded by the tegument, which is bounded by the viral envelope (Figure 3.1). The envelope is derived from the nuclear membrane of the infected cell. Virally encoded glycoprotein spikes protrude from the surface of the envelope[3]. These glycoproteins are important in the pathogenesis, being the targets of many of the antiviral immune responses as well as facilitating entry into permissive cells[4-6].

The genome of HSV-1 has recently been completely sequenced[7] and shown to consist of approximately 152 kilobase pairs comprising some 72 genes encoding 70 distinct proteins. The genome consists of two covalently linked unique regions, the long (UL) and short (US) regions each bounded by short inverted repeat sequences. Recombination occurs, leading to inversion of the unique sequences and the production of four isomeric forms of the genome that are normally present in equimolar concentrations. In latent infections within neurones, the genome structure is different from the linear unit length genome found in the virions. The latent genome is shorter, with the ends missing, suggesting that the virus may be in a circular or highly concatemerized form, and may or may not be integrated into the host DNA[8,9].

24

REPLICATION OF HSV

The replication cycle of HSV within permissive cells is relatively short, with infectious virus being detected 5–6 hours post-infection (pi) and cell lysis occurring 18–20 hours pi. After entry into a permissive cell, the virus uncoats and travels to the nucleus where viral DNA synthesis and assembly of virions occur. Replication proceeds in a series of steps, each producing characteristic proteins that may be recognized by the host immune system. The immediate early genes are first transcribed and their products initiate transcription of the early genes. Products of the early genes downregulate transcription of the immediate early genes and promote transcription of the late genes. Late gene products in turn downregulate transcription of the early genes.

HSV is a comparatively unselective virus and will productively infect a variety of cell types from a number of mammalian species both *in vitro* and *in vivo*. In addition, HSV can abortively infect various other cell types, including those of the monocyte/macrophage lineage that are involved in both natural and specific immune responses. Although no replicating virus results from such an infection, cellular function is disrupted, which may have important implications in disease pathogenesis. In addition, HSV has been reported to downregulate the expression of major histocompatibility complex (MHC) class I cell surface proteins in infected cells[10]. Since MHC class I determinants are the restriction elements used by most cytotoxic T lymphocytes, this may affect the efficiency of recognition and lysis of infected target cells by the immune system.

HSV GLYCOPROTEINS

Many of the proteins coded for by HSV have been characterized and functions have been ascribed to several of them (reviewed in refs. 4 and 5). Of major imortance from the immunopathological viewpoint are the viral glycoproteins that are found in both the virion envelope and the membranes of infected cells and which are the main antigenic determinants seen by the immune system (reviewed in ref. 6). These glycoproteins are implicated in adsorption to and entry of virus into cells, and may well have other important functions in the virus life cycle.

Six distinct HSV glycoproteins (gps) are currently recognized: gB, gC, gD, gE, gG and gH[5]. To date, gH has only been described in HSV-1. The gps are synthesized at specific times during the replication cycle, gD and gE being detectable earliest, followed by gB, which is in turn followed by gC and gG[4]. Virus assembly occurs within the nucleus of the infected cells, with budding through the nuclear membrane, and it is at this stage that the envelope gps are acquired. Viral envelope gps are also detectable in intracellular membranes and at the cell surface. It is of particular immunopathological interest that gE has receptor activity for the Fc portion of immunoglobulin molecules and that the gC of HSV-1 (but not HSV-2) acts as a receptor for the activated third component of the complement system, C3b. Binding of C3b to cell membranes triggers the assembly of the lytic complex of the complement cascade and suggests that gC of HSV-1 may be involved in cell lysis and release of virions, particularly as it is only produced late on in the replication cycle.

SPECIFIC IMMUNE RESPONSES TO HSV

It would be impossible to do justice to the enormous literature on this topic, which has been extensively reviewed recently[1,5,6].

Antibodies are raised in both natural and experimental infections to all the gps, but no neutralizing antibodies have yet been described against gC. The presence of neutralizing antibody is not protective against latent infection, since those individuals who suffer from the greatest frequency of recrudescent lesions have the highest titres. Also, immunosuppressed individuals may suffer from extensive recrudescence even if they are antibody positive and HSV encephalitis has been described in individuals who were previously antibody-positive[2]. Antibody may, however, be protective against secondary infection with a different strain of virus and may play some role in preventing systemic spread of HSV following recrudescences. Thus, for the purposes of vaccine design, the ability to induce antibody is not a sufficiently stringent criterion for selection.

The important immune responses for clearance of virus and possibly prevention of latency establishment and recrudescence have been shown to be those of the cell-mediated immune system[11]. Transfer of T lymphocytes from immune to naive animals has been shown to be protective in a number of systems, including transfer to the athymic nude mouse, to neonatally thymectomized mice, to lethally irradiated mice and to animals treated with cyclophosphamide and antilymphocyte serum[1], underlining the importance of these cells in controlling HSV infections. Both delayed-hypersensitivity T lymphocyte responses (DH) and cytotoxic T lymphocytes (Tc cells) have been shown to be important in the clearance of primary experimental infections[1]. In both experimental and natural infections, recrudescence has been reported to be accompanied by a transient suppression of specific cell-mediated immune responses to HSV[12,13]. Schrier et al.[14] reported that suppression of DH to HSV in a mouse model resulted in concomitant suppression of transferable T cell protection against lethal infection in naive syngeneic animals. In human HSV infections, Tc cells have been reported to recognize gD and gB[15] and in murine experimental models Tc that recognize gC[16] have been described. DH responses have been reported against gB, gD and gC[17,18].

Obviously, the immune responses to any pathogen are many and varied, and are in a complex balance with each other. Thus, it is unfair to state categorically that one response is important and another irrelevant when both may contribute to protective immunity — possibly more importantly — also to any subsequent immunopathology associated with a particular infection. All these factors have to be considered in designing therapeutic approaches to HSV induced disease.

HSV INFECTIONS IN HUMANS

Herpes simplex virus is a common pathogen in human populations, causing a variety of diseases[19]. The virus is present in the vesicle fluid of cutaneous lesions[20], saliva[21], and also tears[22] when the eye is involved. A new individual is infected by contact with these secretions, although frequently no clinical disease is immediately apparent[20]. Such infections are common as shown by the high proportion of the population (50–80%) that has antibodies to HSV, documenting previous infection[19].

There are fundamental differences between primary and recrudescent disease. Primary disease is produced when the host first encounters HSV. The disease depends on the site of inoculation. Serotype 1 HSV usually produces gingivostomatitis or blepharoconjunctivitis as primary disease, whereas serotype 2 causes balanitis or cervicitis[19]. A characteristic of HSV is that despite an immunological response by the host, the virus is able to persist (establish latency) and to reappear and produce recrudescent disease in some individuals. Latency has recently been reviewed by Blyth[23], and Wildy et al.[24]. Recrudescence takes the form of genital sores for HSV serotype 2, and cold sores (herpes labialis) or eye disease for serotype 1.

Once latency has been established, recrudescent disease is due to virus that is always identical from episode to episode, as judged by DNA restriction endonuclease analysis[25]. The isolation of HSV from nerve ganglia provides evidence for the site of latency[26], although evidence is mounting that after ocular herpetic infection the virus may be able to persist in ocular tissue[27–33], possibly in a state identical to that in neural latency (refs. 34 and 35, and Claoué et al., manuscript in preparation). Ocular recrudescent disease does not require ocular primary infection, as spread may occur via neural pathways to infect ganglia "from within" — the "back-door" route[36,37]. However, it has been observed that "To the eye, the menace of the virus-laden kiss is heightened by the tendency of the labial herpetic to avoid lip-contact and prefer instead cheek or brow"[38] — thus the likelihood of a primary ocular infection is increased.

HSV-INDUCED EYE DISEASE IN HUMANS

Herpetic eye disease is frequently seen by clinical ophthalmologists. This is mainly recrudescent disease[39].

Primary herpetic eye disease represents approximately 5% of all cases of herpetic eye disease[40]. It consists of an ulcerative blepharitis with a follicular conjunctivitis. Keratitis similar to that seen in recrudescent disease may develop. One fifth of all follicular conjunctivitis may be primary ocular HSV[41]. The disease now occurs predominantly in adolescents and young adults[42], whereas, previously, younger age groups predominated[43]. The incidence of corneal involvement in primary herpetic eye disease appears to have fallen from 50%[38] to 17%[42]. Both primary and recrudescent disease tends to be more severe in atopic individuals[39,44].

27

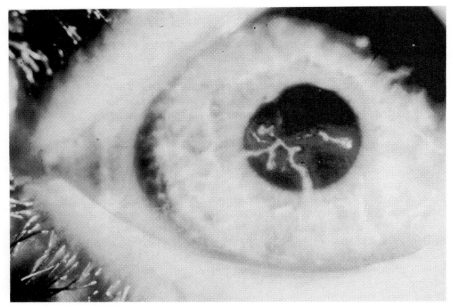

Figure 3.2 Photograph of dendritic ulcer of cornea; this particular case clearly shows the branching of the epithelial lesion due to adherent mucus.

The incidence of recrudescent eye disease is not known, but it has been estimated that 0.05% of the population suffers from herpetic eye disease[45]. Approximately 300 000 patients are diagnosed annually in the USA[46]. These two figures show approximately a fourfold discrepancy, and further epidemiological research in this area is clearly required.

Recrudescent disease occurs in an older age group, with a peak incidence at 40 years and with an overall male preponderance of 2:1[40]. Bilateral (but not necessarily synchronous) disease is found in 6% of patients[47].

Further recrudescences will occur in 40–60% of patients[40,48,49] between 1 and 47 years after the presenting episode. Males are more likely than females to have further recrudescences[50]. Half the patients will retain normal visual acuities but 17% will be reduced to 6/18 or worse[40].

The commonest form of recrudescent ocular disease is keratitis. Clinically, this may involve any or all the three layers of the cornea (the surface epithelium, the stroma, or the endothelium). The nomenclature of herpetic keratitis is often rather loose, particularly the term "stromal keratitis". Classification by pathogenesis would be ideal, but is not possible yet. Reference is frequently made to that layer of the cornea that appears most involved. Other ocular structures may also be involved, with blepharitis, canaliculitis, conjunctivitis, or uveitis occurring either in isolation or in conjunction with keratitis. Although more common in primary herpetic eye disease, an angular blepharitis[51] or ulcerative marginal blepharitis[52] may be produced in recurrent disease. HSV conjunctivitis is most commonly seen in primary disease, but may rarely be the sole manifestation of recurrent disease.

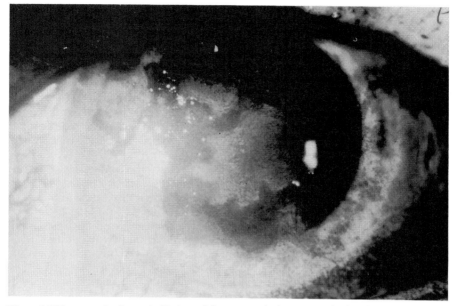

Figure 3.3 Photograph of amoeboid ulcer of the cornea; the large area of epithelial loss has been darkly stained with rose bengal

Conjunctival injection may be association with punched-out ulcers and a papillary or follicular response[53-55].

Epithelial ulceration in dendritic (Figure 3.2) and amoeboid (Figure 3.3) keratititis is accepted to be due to viral replication[56], and viral antigens can be demonstrated in corneal scrapes from such patients[57].

Metaherpetic ulceration results in a sterile, round corneal ulcer with grey sharp edges that is slow to heal[58]. It was originally described by Gundersen[22], who found the incidence to be 19.5%; Sundmacher[59] reported that 32% of his patients developed this condition. With the use of less-toxic antiviral drugs the condition has become rare, and Wilhelmus[50] found only 0.7% of patients affected. Metaherpetic ulceration occurs when HSV or the host response damages the epithelial basement membrane, thereby preventing cell adhesion over the damaged area[39]. Other factors may contribute to its development, including corneal anaesthesia and alterations in the tear film constituents (see ref. 60 for a full discussion).

Ulceration of the cornea from any cause, if persistent, will result in an influx of inflammatory cells[61]. Thus, any purely epithelial disease (such as dendritic ulceration) can result in an epiphenomenon of stromal disease[61,62]. Usually, such stromal disease consists merely of a localized superficial stromal infiltrate below and immediately adjacent to the ulcerated area. In addition, epithelial herpetic ulcers can become secondarily infected by bacteria[49].

Disciform oedema is a well-described clinical entity consisting of a patch of circular stromal oedema associated with an anterior uveitis. Keratic

29

precipitates are usually found on the underlying endothelium. The corneal oedema frequently clears with minimal or no treatment and there are no reports of histological studies of the acute disease. However, a number of reports have been made on the histology of the quiescent scarred stage in those eyes that required enucleation or penetrating keratoplasty[63-65]. These reports are relatively disparate, and obviously refer to atypical cases of disciform oedema. All these authors comment on the mixed nature of the inflammatory cell populations to be found in the cornea, including polymorphonuclear leukocytes, lymphocytes and plasma cells. The pathogenesis is thus obscure, although from the histology it has been suggested that type IV hypersentivity is important[66].

In contrast, Vannas et al.[67] have suggested that HSV may directly invade the corneal endothelium from a herpetic uveitis. They propose that any corneal scarring is due to persisting oedema and to immunological and inflammatory responses to the HSV-induced "endotheliitis". At present, there is no good evidence to support any specific mechanism suggested as the cause of disciform oedema in humans. However, an excellent study by Collum, Logan, and Ravenscroft[68] has shown unequivocally that patients treated with a combination of topical steroid and acyclovir respond significantly better than patients receiving topical placebo and acyclovir. The beneficial effect of steroid indirectly supports the concept that the host response contributes significantly to the genesis of the clinical disease, but offers no other insight into whether the mechanisms are immunological or purely inflammatory.

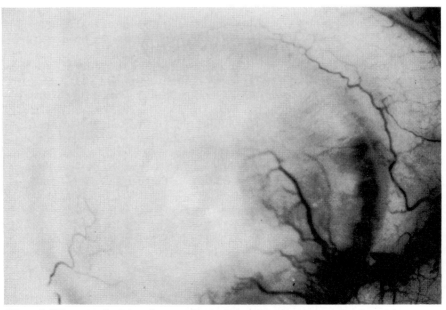

Figure 3.4 Photograph of chronic stromal herpetic keratitis. Note the opacification of the cornea, concealing iris detail (compare with Figures 3.2 and 3.3), and the ingrowth of blood vessels

Chronic herpetic stromal keratitis may occur with or without epithelial ulceration. This disease is principally characterized by its chronicity and generalized stromal opacification (Figure 3.4). An anterior uveitis is usual, but may be obscured by corneal opacification. Long-standing disease leads to the growth of leashes of corneal new vessels in the stroma. This is a condition that all too frequently leads to corneal blindness requiring penetrating keratoplasty, which regrettably is not always successful in producing visual rehabilitation owing to allograft rejection, recurrent disease, or optical problems[39]. This is the major clinical problem in human herpetic eye disease.

Anterior uveitis in herpetic eye disease is divided into two types[69,70]. The first is a mild iritis seen in all cases of epithelial keratitis. It is postulated that this occurs as an irritative reaction mediated by prostaglandins[70-72]. The second type is more severe[73], with raised intraocular pressure[67,72,74] and focal iris necrosis particularly in the region of the sphincter[69,74]. This usually occurs with stromal keratitis, but may occur in isolation[73]. The diagnosis may be confirmed by surgically tapping the aqueous humour from the anterior chamber of the eye, which may reveal viral antigens in cells[75,76], viral particles visible by electron microscopy[76,77], or isolation of infectious virus[78-80]. It seems likely that HSV is capable of invading the anterior uvea producing a productive infection and a severe anterior uveitis. Rarely, HSV may produce a posterior uveitis[81,82] or panuveitis[80]. This also appears to be due to replicating virus.

ANIMAL MODELS OF HSV DISEASE

Attempts have been made to produce experimental disease that mimics that seen in humans. Although they have been successful in producing disease, the nomenclature of human disease has been applied in a rather loose fashion, with the result that workers using the same model have variously referred to the disease as "disciform oedema", "stromal necrosis", or "interstitial keratitis". This has created much confusion.

Animal models have been used widely to investigate the pathogenesis of HSV-induced disease[1,83]. The use of such models takes advantage of the non-selective nature of HSV which causes clinical symptoms in a variety of mammalian species as well as its natural host, humans. There is no doubt that animal models have provided a wealth of information about the various pathologies associated with HSV infection, but their usefulness is limited by (1) the degree to which the outcome of natural infection can be mimicked, and by (2) the extent to which the host reponse in any particular model reflects that of the natural host.

The most commonly used animal models have been the rabbit, the guinea pig and the laboratory mouse, all of which have been used to study epidermal and systemic infections with both HSV serotypes. The rabbit and mouse models have also been extensively used for the study of ocular HSV infections, reviewed by Kumel et al.[84].

Several interacting factors must be considered when selecting a model of a particular HSV-induced disease state in order to build up a complete picture of the pathogenic events occurring. These include the following:

31

Virus-related factors

Different strains and isolates of virus have been shown to cause different patterns of disease in the same host species (reviewed by Marsden[5]). These differences may be due to mutations in viral thymidine kinase genes[85], variations in the antigenic structure of the gB, gC, or gD[84], or alterations in parts of the genome of as yet unknown function such as the region between 0.71 and 0.83 map units, which was shown by Centifanto–Fitzgerald et al.[86] to be involved in patterns of ocular disease in a mouse model. However, it must be considered that the use of laboratory-adapted strains of virus may not give a true picture of the pathogenic effects induced by wild-type viruses.

Host-related factors

Host-related factors include natural resistance to HSV infection, specific immune responses to HSV and the status of the host immune system at the time of primary or recrudescent infection (maturity, immunosuppression, concurrent infection with other pathogens). Natural resistance is important in determining susceptibility to HSV infection; this has been studied extensively in mouse models, where a wide variety of generating inbred strains are available. Lopez[87] demonstrated that strains could be described as highly susceptible, highly resistant, or intermediately susceptible to a given intraperitoneal inoculum of HSV. Genetic factors were involved but these were not related to the species MHC antigens. The same patterns of resistance/ susceptibility are seen in murine ocular HSV infection[88]. Foster et al.[89] reported that HSV keratitis was linked to the immunoglobulin IgH-1 locus, although there was no evidence that antibody as such was involved. Other authors have suggested that differences in susceptibility may be due to the ability of virus to infect cells of various strains[88]. Natural killer cell efficiency has also been implicated in natural resistance to HSV infection[90]. Specific immune responses to HSV have been described above and are undoubtedly of paramount importance in containing HSV infection but, as will be considered later, may also contribute significantly to the degree and type of associated damaging pathology. The ability to mount an immune response to HSV and the type of response generated depend upon the status of the individual immune system at the time of infection. Lack of immunological maturity contributes to the disseminated life-threatening disease caused by neonatal exposure to HSV. Those who are therapeutically or genetically immunosuppressed may also suffer severe disseminated HSV disease as do certain atopic patients. Transient local immunosuppression at the site of primary infection has also been shown to alter both the nature of the immune response generated and the pattern of subsequent disease manifestations[91,92]. Concurrent infection with other pathogens may cause recrudescence of latent infection, possibly through deleterious effects on the host immune system.

ANIMAL MODELS OF OCULAR HERPES SIMPLEX INFECTION

Many animal models have been specifically developed to study the pathology of ocular HSV infection, the most widely used being the rabbit and the mouse[83,93]. Whilst there is no doubt that the simple fact of infection of ocular tissue leads to damage depending upon viral factors outlined above and that the latent infection may even be established in ocular cells[32,35,94], in recent years much attention has been focused on the role of the immune response in controlling and contributing to the pathology of ocular HSV infection.

This research has demonstrated the importance of the specific immune response in localizing ocular HSV infection, since athymic mice infected by corneal scarification die from disseminated infection[95,96]. However, the roles of the various effector immune responses in recovery are not yet fully understood. T-cell responses have been reported as responsible for recovery from ocular infection[97,98] as have antibody responses[99]. Treatment with HSV-specific monoclonal antibodies has been reported to protect against ocular disease[100] as has previous immunization with an apathogenic strain of virus[101].

On the other hand, the various effector mechanisms of the immune response have also been reported as contributing to the actual pathology of ocular HSV infection. Jordan et al.[102] reported that corneal infection in a mouse model was diminished by depletion of B lymphocytes with mortality being reduced from 89% to 42%. Russell et al.[96] showed that athymic mice developed encephalitis and disseminated HSV infection after corneal inoculation, but did not develop stromal lesions, whereas their euthymic littermates developed only localized stromal lesions, indicating that T lymphocytes were important for containment of infection, but also contributed to the development of stromal disease.

To understand the apparent paradox between the protective and pathogenic aspects of the immune response involves an appreciation of the fact that although the immune response is essentially unlimited in the number of foreign antigens to which it can respond, it is fairly limited in the number of specific effector mechanisms it has at its disposal, i.e. antibody production, T lymphocyte cytotoxicity, and delayed hypersensitivity (DH). Generally speaking, antigens encountered at the body's surface generate initially a DH response and may or may not elicit cytotoxic T lymphocyte and antibody responses subsequently. Whereas DH is an efficient method of clearing antigen from localized peripheral sites, it nevertheless involves a degree of local tissue damage that may be of little overall importance to the epidermis but may have far more severe pathological consequences in more specialized tissues such as the eye and the lungs. Similarly, antibody-mediated or T lymphocyte cytotoxicity of infected cells in such specialized tissues, if allowed to proceed unchecked, may cause an unacceptable degree of local damage. To control this to some extent, the host defence of these tissues has evolved such that there is a rapid generation of specific suppression of DH responses, which has been reported in the eye for HSV infection[103] and alloantigen responses[104]. This suppression appears to result from altered antigen presentation within

33

these tissues, which may be due to the lack of Langerhans cells (the normal epidermal antigen-presenting cells) reported in the corneal epithelium[105]. More probably, there is an alteration in the balance between the induction of DH and its suppression in these tissues that would ideally allow for effective control of infection in the absence of immunopathology. Unfortunately, in some individuals the balance is not perfect and immunopathological damage does occur. The use of animal models may allow a better understanding of the immunological mechanisms involved and hopefully this will lead to effective methods of externally modulating the antiviral immune response and the possibility of vaccination regimes to prevent the appearance of primary and/or recrudescent disease.

HSV AND IMMUNOPATHOLOGY IN THE HUMAN EYE

The majority of severe herpetic keratitits occurs in patients after several previous milder episodes. There have therefore been several occasions on which antigens have been presented to the immune system.

Why does recrudescent disease occur? Since recrudescent disease occurs in the presence of serum antibody, it is clear that this is not protective. The mechanism of control of latency in humans is not known, but recently evidence has been presented showing antigen-specific reduced cell-mediated immunity to HSV at the time of recrudescent disease for herpes labialis[106,107], genital herpes[108], and ocular herpes[109,110]. Hendricks and Sugar[111] have presented data suggesting that a specific population of NK cells able to lyse target cells displaying HSV antigens is reduced in patients suffering recurrent disease. This was due to active suppression by a T suppressor subpopulation. Futhermore, the prevalence of cytomegalovirus (a related human herpes virus) retinitis in patients with acquired immunodeficiency syndrome (AIDS) again supports the controlling role of the immune system.

The pathophysiology of chronic stromal keratitis in humans is not well understood. There have been no histological studies of early untreated cases. Light-microscopic studies on late scarred cases requiring enucleation or penetrating keratoplasty have documented the presence of predominantly PMN infiltration[63,112,113] or a mixed inflammatory population[114-116] with necrotic stromal lamellae[63], fibroblastic activity[63], a duplication of Descemet's membrane[117], and a severely abnormal endothelium[112].

Early reports suggest that many of the lymphocytes in atypical cases of severe stromal keratitis with stromal necrosis may bear the same antigens as cytotoxic T cells[118,119]. In these studies, inflammatory cells were eluted from corneal buttons removed at the time of emergency ("à chaud") penetrating keratoplasty. These results provide support for the hypothesis that in certain circumstances, cell-mediated immune mechanisms may play a pathogenic role in the development of human herpetic keratitis.

It is known that viral antigens are present on keratocytes, as shown by immunofluorescence[114] and immunoelectron microscopy[113]. Furthermore, many authors have documented complete or incomplete viral particles in keratocytes in at least some specimens[112-115,120] and thus HSV antigens can be presented either in particulate or cell membrane-associated form. The former would be capable of forming fixed immune complexes in the cornea, and have been proposed as the cause of the so-called "immune ring" of opacification occasionally seen in the corneas of patients with herpetic eye disease. There is no direct human evidence to support these contentions.

Further circumstantial evidence for the role of the immune system in human herpetic eye disease is the severity of such disease in atopic individuals. The underlying mechanisms are not known, but clearly a genetic predisposition to production of an abnormal immunological response is capable of enchancing pathogenic mechanisms in these patients. There do not appear to have been any reports of herpes simplex eye disease in congenital or acquired immunodeficiency states, although were they to occur such "experiments of nature" might provide valuable information.

CONCLUSIONS

Whilst it is clear that immunopathology occurs in experimental ocular herpetic infection, unequivocal evidence for immune-mediated tissue damage in human herpetic eye disease does not exist. There is, however, mounting circumstantial evidence that such pathogenic mechanisms are operating. Clearly, further research is required.

Although some authorities believe that the incidence of severe human herpetic keratitis is falling owing to better management and more effective antiviral therapy, a recent study has shown no fall in the proportion of penetrating keratoplasties performed for herpetic keratitis (Claoué, Flacon and Shilling, manuscript in preparation). It would seem desirable, therefore, for further basic research on immune modulation to be coupled to a greater understanding of pathogenic mechanisms in the human cornea, with a view to sparing future generations of patients from the unpleasant, mutilating, and recurrent effects of herpes simplex virus keratitis.

Acknowledgements

C. C. acknowledges the encouragement of and helpful discussions with Mr M. G. Falcon and Miss K. E. Stevenson during the preparation of this manuscript.

S. H. is grateful to Dr M. Norval, Mr D. Yirrell and Mrs J. Maingay for many useful discussions and to the Medical Research Council of Great Britain for financial support.

We are also grateful to Dr I. Christie of the Department of Virology at St Thomas' Hospital for supplying the electron micrograph shown in Figure 3.1.

References

1. Widly, P. H. and Gell, P. G. H. (1983). The host response to herpes simplex virus. *Br. Med. Bull.*, **41**, 86–91

2. Anon. (1985). Prevention and control of herpesvirus diseases. *Bull. World Health Org.*, **63**, 427–44
3. Stannard, L. M., Fuller, A. O. and Spear, P. G. (1987). Herpes simplex virus glycoproteins associated with different morphological entities projecting from the virion envelope. *J. Gen. Virol.*, **68**, 715–25
4. Spear, P. G. (1985). Glycoproteins specified by herpes simplex virus. In Roizman, B. (ed.) *The Herpesviruses* Vol. 3, pp. 315–56. (New York: Plenum Press)
5. Marsden, H. S. (1987). Herpes simplex virus glycoproteins and pathogenesis. *Soc. Gen. Microbiol. Symposium* **40**, 259–88. (Cambridge: Cambridge University Press)
6. Maingay, J. P., Norval, M. and Howie, S. (1988). The immune response to glycoproteins of the herpes simplex virus. *Microbiol. Sci.*, **5**, 211–15
7. McGeoch, D. J., Dalyrymple, M. A., Davison, A. J., Dolan, A., Frame, M. C., McNab, D., Perry, L. J., Scott, J. E. and Taylor, P. (1988). The complete DNA sequence of the long unique region in the genome of simplex virus type 1. *J. Gen. Virol.*, **69**, 1531–74
8. Rock, D. L. and Fraser, N. W. (1983). Detection of HSV-1 genome in central nervous system of latently infected mice. *Nature*, **302**, 523–25
9. Efstathiou, S., Minson, A. C., Field, H. J., Anderson, J. R. and Wildy,P. (1986). Detection of herpes simplex virus-specific DNA sequences in latently infected mice and in humans. *J. Virol.*, **57**, 446–55
10. Jennings, S. R., Rice, P. L., Kloszewski, E. D., Anderson, R. W., Thompson, D. L. and Tevethia, S. S. (1985). Effect of herpes simplex virus types 1 and 2 on surface expression of class 1 major histocompatibility complex antigens on infected cells. *J. Virol.*, **56**, 757–66
11. Oakes, J. E. (1975). Role for cell mediated immunity in the resistance of mice to subcutaneous herpes simplex infection. *Infect. Immun.*, **12**, 166–72
12. Sheridan, J. F., Donnenberg, A. D., Aurelian, L. and Elpern, D. J. (1982). Immunity to herpes simplex virus type 2 IV. Impaired lymphokine production during recrudescence correlates with an imbalance in T cell subsets. *J. Immunol.*, **129**, 326–31
13. Sheridan, J. F., Beck, M., Smith, C. C. and Aurelian, L. (1987). Reactivation of herpes simplex virus is associated with production of a low molecular weight factor that inhibits lymphokine activity in vitro. *J. Immunol.*, **138**, 1234–9
14. Schrier, R. D., Ishioka, G. Y., Pizer, L. I. and Moorhead, J. W. (1985). Delayed hypersensitivity and immune protection against herpes simplex virus: suppressor T cells that regulate the induction of delayed type hypersensitivity T cells also regulate the induction of protective T cells. *J. Immunol.*, **134**, 2889–93
15. Zarling, J. M., Moran, P. A., Burke, R. L., Pachl, C., Berman, P. W. and Lasky, L. A. (1986). Human cytotoxic T cell clones directed against herpes simplex virus infected cells IV. Recognition and activation by clonal glycoproteins gB and gD. *J. Immunol.*, **136**, 4669–73
16. Rosenthal, K. L., Smiley, K., South, S. and Johnson, D. C. (1987). Cells expressing herpes simplex virus glycoprotein gC, but not gB, gD, or gE are recognised by murine virus specific cytotoxic T lymphocytes. *J. Virol.*, **61**, 2438–47
17. Glorioso, J. C., Szczesiul, M. S., Marlin, S. D. and Levine, M. (1983). Inhibition of glycosylation of herpes simplex virus glycoproteins: identification of antigenic and immunogenic partially glycosylated glycoproteins on the cell surface membrane. *Virology*, **126**, 1–18
18. Schrier, R. D., Pizer, L. and Moorhead, J. W. (1983). Type-specific delayed hypersensitivity and protective immunity induced by isolated herpes simplex virus glycoprotein. *J. Immunol.*, **130**, 1413
19. Nahmias, A. J. and Josey, W. E. (1976). Epidemiology of herpes simplex viruses. In Evans, A. S. (ed.). *Viral Infections of Humans, Epidemiology and Control*. (London: Wiley)
20. Robinson, T. W. E. and Heath, R. B. (1983). *Virus Diseases and the Skin*, pp. 56–70. (London: Churchill Livingstone)
21. Buddingh, G. J., Schrum, D. I., Lanier, J. C. and Guidry, D. J. (1953). Studies of the natural history of herpes simplex infections. *Paediatrics*, **11**, 595–610
22. Gundersen, T. (1936). Herpes cornea: with special reference to its treatment with strong solutions of iodine. *Arch. Ophthalmol.*, **15**, 225–49
23. Blyth, W. A. (1985). Latency and recurrence in herpes simplex virus infection. In Easty D. L. (ed.) *Viral Disease of the Eye*, pp. 83–92. (London: Lloyd-Luke)

24. Wildy, P., Field, H. J. and Nash, A. A. (1982). Classical herpes latency revisited. In Mahy, B. W. J., Minson, A. C. and Darby, G. K. (eds.) *Virus Persistence*, pp. 133–167. (Cambridge: Cambridge University Press)

25. Asbell, P. A., Centifanto-Fitzgerald, Y. M., Chandler, J. W. and Kaufman, H. E. (1984). Analysis of viral DNA in isolates from patients with recurrent herpetic keratitis. *Invest. Ophthalmol. Vis. Sci.*, **25**, 951–4

26. Tullo, A. B., Shimeld, C., Easty, D. L. and Darville, J. M. (1983). Distribution of latent herpes simplex virus infection in human trigeminal ganglion. *Lancet*, **1**, 353

27. Shimeld, C., Tullo, A. B., Easty, D. L. and Thomsitt, J. (1982). Isolation of herpes simplex virus from the cornea in chronic stromal keratitis. *Br. J. Ophthalmol.*, **66**, 643–7

28. Tullo, A. B., Easty, D. L., Stirling, P. E. and Darville, J. M. (1985). Isolation of herpes simplex virus from corneal discs of patients with chronic stromal keratitis. *Trans. Opthalmol. Soc. U.K.*, **104**, 159–65

29. Coupes, D., Klapper, R. E., Cleator, G. M., Bailey, A. S. and Tullo, A. B. (1986). Herpes simplex virus in chronic human stromal keratitis. *Curr. Eye Res.*, **5**, 735–8

30. Cook, S. D., Aitken, D. A., Loeffler, K. U. and Brown, S. M. (1986). Herpes simplex virus in the cornea: an ultrastructural study on viral reactivation. *Trans. Ophthalmol. Soc. U.K.*, **105**, 634–41

31. Cook, S. D. and Brown, S. M. (1966). Herpes simplex virus type 1 persistence and latency in cultured rabbit corneal epithelial cells, keratocytes, and endothelial cells. *Br. J. Ophthalmol.*, **70**, 642–50

32. Cook, S. D. and Brown, S. M. (1987). Herpes simplex virus type 1 latency in rabbit corneal cells in vitro: reactivation and recombination following intratypic superinfection of long term cultures. *J. Gen. Virol.*, **68**, 813–24

33. Abghari, S. Z. and Stulting, R. D. (1988). Recovery of herpes simplex virus from ocular tissues of latently infected inbred mice. *Invest. Ophthalmol. Vis. Sci.*, **29**, 239–43

34. Easty, D. L., Shimeld, C., Claoué, C. M. P. and Menage, M. (1987). Herpes simplex virus isolation in chronic stromal keratitis; human and laboratory studies. *Curr. Eye Res.*, **6**(1), 69–74

35. Claoué, C. M. P., Esty, D. L., Blyth, W. A. and Hill, T. J. (1987). Does herpes simplex virus establish latency in the eye of the mouse? *Eye*, **1**(4), 525–8

36. Tullo, A. B. (1982). Mechanisms of latent and recurrent ocular infection with herpes simplex virus. *M.D. Thesis*, University of Bristol.

37. Tullo, A. B., Easty, D. L., Hill, T. J. and Blyth W. A. (1982). Ocular herpes simplex and the establishment of latent infection. *Trans. Ophthalmol. Soc. U.K.*, **102**, 15–18

38. Jones, B. (1959). The management of ocular herpes. *Trans. Ophthalmol. Soc. U.K.*, **79**, 425–37

39. Easty, D. L. (ed.) (1985). *Viral Disease of the Eye*. (London: Lloyd-Luke)

40. Norn, M. S. (1970). Dendritic (herpetic) keratitis: 2. Follow up examination of corneal opacity. *Acta Ophthalmol.*, **48**, 214–26

41. Wishart, P. K., James, C., Wishart, M. S. and Darougar, S. (1984). Prevalence of acute conjunctivitis caused by chlamydia, adenovirus, and herpes simplex virus in an ophthalmic casualty department. *Br. J. Ophthalmol.*, **68**, 653–5

42. Darougar, S., Wishart, M. S. and Viswalingam, N. D. (1985). Epidemiological and clinical features of primary herpes simplex virus ocular infection. *Br. J. Ophthalmol.*, **69**, 2–6

43. Patterson, A. and Jones, B. R. (1967). The management of ocular herpes. *Trans. Ophthalmol. Soc. U.K.*, **87**, 59–84

44. Wilhelmus, K. R., Falcon, M. G. and Jones, B. R. (1981). Bilateral herpetic keratitis. *Br. J. Ophthalmol.*, **65**, 385–7

45. Norn, M. S. (1970). Dendritic (herpetic) keratitis: I. Incidence, seasonal variations, recurrence rate, visual impairment, therapy. *Acta Ophthalmol.*, **48**, 91–107

46. Pavan-Langston, D. (1975). Diagnosis and management of herpes simplex ocular infection. *Int. Ophthalmol. Clin.*, **15**, 19–35

47. Tullo, A. B. (1985). Herpes simplex keratitis: latent and recurrent infection. In Easty, D. L. and Smolin, G. (eds.) *External Eye Disease*, pp. 133–53. (London: Butterworths)

48. Carroll, J. M., Martola, E.-L., Laibson, P. R. and Dohlman, C. H. (1967). The recurrence of herpetic keratitis following idoxuridine therapy. *Am. J. Ophthalmol.*, **63**(1), 103–7

49. Wilhelmus, K. R. (1982). Suppurative corneal ulceration following herpetic keratitis. *Doc.*

Ophthalmol., **53** 17–36

50. Wilhelmus, K. R., Coster, D. J., Falcon, M. G. and Jones, M. C. (1981). Longitudinal analysis of ulcerative herpetic keratitis. In Sundmacher, R. (ed.) *Herpes Eye Disease*, pp. 375. (Munich: J. F. Bergmann Verlag)

51. Jacobiec, F. A., Srinivasan, B. D. and Gamboa, E. T. (1979). Recurrent herpetic angular blepharitis in an adult. *Am. J. Ophthalmol.*, **88**, 744–7

52. Egerer, I. and Stary, A. (1980). Erosive-ulcerative herpes simplex blepharitis. *Arch. Ophthalmol.*, **98**, 1760–3

53. Brown, D. C., Nesburn, A. B., Nauheim, J. S. *et al.* (1969). Recurrent herpes simplex conjunctivitis. *Arch. Ophthalmol.*, **79**, 733–5

54. Nauheim, J. S. (1969). Recurrent herpes simplex conjunctival ulceration. *Arch. Ophthalmol.*, **81**, 592–5

55. Colin, J., Legrignou, A., Baikoff, G. and Chastel, C. (1980). Three cases of dendritic herpetic ulceration of the conjuctiva. *Am. J. Ophthalmol.*, **89**, 608–9

56. O'Day, D. M. and Jones, B. R. (1983). Herpes simplex keratitis. In Duane, T. D. (ed.) *Clinical Ophthalmology*. (Philadelphia: Harper and Row)

57. Collum, L. M. T., Mullaney, J. and Hillery, M. (1986). A suggested rapid test for corneal herpes simplex. *N. Engl. J. Med.*, **314**(4), 245

58. Kaufman, H. E. (1964). Epithelial erosion syndrome: metaherpetic keratitis. *Am. J. Ophthalmol.*, **57**, 983–7

59. Sundmacher, R. and Neumann-Haefelin, D. (1976). Keratitis metaherpetica. Klinische und virologische befunde. *Klin. Mbl. Augenheilk*, **169**, 728–37

60. van Bijsterveld, O. P. and de Koning, E. W. J. (1964). Trophic herpetic corneal ulcers. In Blodi, F. C. (ed.) *Herpes Simplex Infections of the Eye*, pp. 29–45. (London: Churchill Livingstone)

61. Sery, T. W., Richman, M. W. and Nagy, R. M. (1966). Experimental disciform keratitis I. Immune response of the cornea to herpes simplex virus. *J. Allergy*, **86**, 338–51

62. Taktikos, A. and Aurelian, L. (1966). Experimental study of the disease of the corneal stroma caused by herpes simplex virus. *Am. J. Ophthalmol.*, **62**, 1136–41

63. Kimura, S. J. (1962). Herpes simplex uveitis: a clinical and experimental study. *Trans. Am. Ophthalmol. Soc.*, **60**, 440–70

64. Hogan, M. J., Kimura, S. J. and Thygeson, P. (1964). Pathology of herpes simplex kerato-iritis. *Am. J. Ophthalmol.*, **57**, 551–64

65. Teitelbaum, C. S., Streelen, B. W. and Dawson, C. R. (1986). Histopathology of herpes simplex keratouveitis. *Invest. Ophthalmol. Vis. Sci.*, **27**(3), ARVO supplement, p. 47

66. Pavan-Langston, D. (1983). Viral diseases: herpetic diseases. In Smolin, G. and Thoft, R. A. (eds.), *The Cornea — Scientific Foundations and Clinical Practice*, p. 178. (Boston: Little, Brown & Co)

67. Vannas, A., Ahonen, R. and Mukitie, J. (1983). Corneal endothelium in herpetic keratouveitis. *Arch. Ophthalmol.*, **101**, 913–15

68. Collum, L. M. T., Logan, P. and Ravenscroft, T. (1983). Acyclovir (Zovirax) in herpetic disciform keratitis. *Br. J. Ophthalmol.* **67**, 115–18

69. Waterworth, D. (1967). Herpes simplex iridocyclitis. *Trans. Ophthalmol. Soc. Aust.* **26**, 120–2

70. Dawson, C. R. and Togni, B. (1976). Herpes simplex eye infections: clinical manifestations, pathogenesis and management. *Surv. Ophthalmol.*, **21**(2), 121–35

71. Sears, M. L., Neufeld, A. H. and Jampol, L. M. (1973). Prostaglandins. *Invest. Ophthalmol. Vis. Sci.*, **12**, 161–4

72. O'Connor, G. R. (1976). Recurrent herpes simplex uveitis in humans. *Surv. Ophthalmol.*, **21**, 165–70

73. Thygeson, P., Hogan, M. J. and Kimura, S. J. (1957). Observations on uveitis associated with viral disease. *Trans. Am. Ophthalmol. Soc.*, **55**, 333–52

74. Wilhelmus, K. R., Falcon, M. G. and Jones, B. R. (1981). Herpetic iridocyclitis. *Int. Ophthalmol.*, **4**(3), 143–50

75. Patterson, A., Sommerville, R. G. and Jones, B. R. (1968). Herpetic keratouveitis with herpes virus antigen in the anterior chamber. *Trans. Ophthalmol. Soc. U.K.*, **88**, 243–9

76. Kaufman, H. E., Kanai, A. and Ellison, E. D. (1971). Herpetic iritis: Demonstration of virus in the anterior chamber by fluorescent antibody techniques and electron microscopy.

Am. J. Ophthalmol., **71**, 465–9
77. Witmer, R. and Iwanoto, T. (1968). Electron microscope observations of herpes-like particles in the iris. *Arch. Ophthalmol.*, **79**, 331–7
78. Cavara, V. (1954). The role of viruses in the aetiology of uveitis. *Conc. Ophthalmol. Logic.*, **II**, 1232–318
79. Hewson, G. E. (1957). Iritis due to herpes virus. *Irish J. Med. Sci.*, **6**, 372–3
80. Pavan-Langston, D. and Brockhurst, R. J. (1969). Herpes simplex panuveitis. *Arch. Ophthalmol.*, **81**, 783–7
81. Honda, Y., Nakazawa, Y. and Chihara, E. (1983). Necrotising chorioretinitis induced by herpes simplex virus infection in the neonate. *Metab. Paediat. Syst. Ophthalmol.*, **7**, 147–52
82. Gruntzmacher, R. D., Henderson, D., McDonald, P. J. and Coster, D. J. (1983). Herpes simplex chorioretinitis in a healthy adult. *Am. J. Ophthalmol.*, **96**, 788–76
83. Goodpasture, E. W. and Teague, O. (1923). Transmission of the virus of herpes febrilis along nerves in experimentally infected rabbits. *J. Med. Res.*, **44**, 139–84
84. Kumel, G., Kaerner, H. C., Levine, M., Schroder, C. H. and Glorioso, J. C. (1985). Passive immune protection by herpes simplex virus-specific monoclonal antibodies and monoclonal antibody resistant mutants altered in pathogenicity. *J. Virol.*, **56**, 930–7
85. Field, H. J. and Wildy, P. (1978). The pathogenicity of thymidine kinase deficient mutants of herpes simplex virus in mice. *J. Hygiene*, **81**, 267–77
86. Centifanto-Fitzgerald, Y. M., Varnell, E. D. and Kaufman, H. E. (1985). Ocular disease pattern induced by herpes simplex virus is genetically determined by a specific region of viral DNA. *J. Exp. Med.*, **155**, 475–89
87. Lopez, C. (1975). Genetics of natural resistance to herpes virus infections in mice. *Nature*, **258**, 152–3
88. Pepose, J. S. and Whittum-Hudson, J. A. (1987). An immunogenetic analysis of resistance to herpes simplex virus retinitis in inbred strains of mice. *Invest. Ophthalmol. Vis. Sci.*, **28**, 1549–552
89. Foster, C. S., Tsai, Y., Monroe, J. G., Campbell, R., Cestari, M., Werzig, R., Knipe, D. and Greene, M. I. (1986). Genetic studies on murine susceptibility to herpes simplex keratitis. *Clin. Immunol. Immunopathol.*, **40**, 313–25
90. Rager-Zisman, B., Quan, P. C., Rosner, M., Moller, J. R. and Bloom, B. R. (1987). Role of NK cells in protection of mice against lethal herpes simplex virus-1 infection. *J. Immunol.*, **138**, 884–8
91. Howie, S. E. M., Norval, M., Maingay, J. and Ross, J. A. (1986). Two phenotypically distinct T cells (Ly1+1– and Ly1-2+) are involved in ultraviolet B light induced suppression of efferent DTH response to HSV *in vivo*. *Immunology*, **58**, 653–8
92. Norval, M., Howie, S. E. M., Ross, J. A. and Maingay, J. P. (1987). A murine model of herpes simplex virus recrudescence. *J. Gen. Virol.*, **68**, 2693–8
93. Hill, T. J. (1987). Ocular pathogenesis of herpes simplex virus. *Curr. Eye Res.*, **6**, 1–7
94. Sabbaga, E. M. H., Pavan-Langston, D., Bean, K. M. and Dunkel, E. C. (1988). Detection of HSV nucleic acid sequences in the cornea during acute and latent ocular disease. *Exp. Eye Res.*, **47**, 545–63
95. Metcalf, J. F., Hamilton, D. S. and Reichert, R. W. (1979). Herpetic keratitis in athymic (nude) mice. *Infect. Immun.*, **26**, 1164–71
96. Russell, R. G., Nasisse, M. P., Larsen, H. S. and Rouse, B. T. (1984). Role of T lymphocytes in the pathogenesis of herpetic stromal keratitis. *Invest. Ophthalmol. Vis. Sci.*, **25**, 938–44
97. Oakes, J. E., Rector, J. T. and Lausch, R. N. (1984). Ly1+ T cells participate in recovery from ocular herpes simplex virus type 1 infection. *Invest. Ophthalmol. Vis. Sci.*, **25**, 188–94
98. Whittum-Hudson, J., Farazdaghi, M. and Prendergast, L. A. (1985). A role for T lymphocytes in preventing experimental herpes simplex virus type-1 induced retinitis. *Invest. Ophthalmol. Vis. Sci.*, **26**, 1524–32
99. Oakes, J. E. and Lausch, R. N. (1981). Role of Fc fragments in antibody mediated recovery from ocular and subcutaneous herpes simplex virus infection. *Infect. Immun.*, **33**, 109–14
100. Metcalf, J. F., Chatterjee, S., Koga, J. and Whitley, R. J. (1988). Protection against herpetic ocular disease by immunotherapy with monoclonal antibodies. *Intervirology*, **29**, 39–49
101. Sandstrom, I. K., Foster, C. S., Wells, P. A., Knipe, D., Caron, L. and Greene, M. I. (1986).

Previous immunisation of mice with herpes simplex virus type-1 strain MP protects against secondary corneal infection. *Clin. Immunol. Immunopathol.*, **40**, 326–34

102. Jordan, C., Boron, F., Dianzani, F., Barber, J. and Stanton, J. (1983). Ocular herpes simplex virus infection is diminished by depletion of B lymphocytes. *J. Immunol.*, **131**, 1554–7

103. Metzger, E. E. and Whittum-Hudson, J. A. (1987). The dichotomy between herpes simplex type-1 induced ocular pathology and systemic immunity. *Invest. Ophthalmol. Vis. Sci.*, **28**, 1533–40

104. Niederkorn, J. Y. and Streilein, J. W. (1983). Alloantigens placed into the anterior chamber of the eye induce specific suppression of delayed type hypersensitivity but normal cytotoxic T lymphocyte and helper T lymphocyte responses. *J. Immunol.*, **131**, 2670–4

105. Peeler, J., Niederkorn, J. and Matoba, A. (1985). Corneal allografts induce cytotoxic T cell but not delayed hypersensitivity responses in mice. *Invest. Ophthalmol. Vis. Sci.*, **26**, 1516–23

106. Wilton, J. M. A., Ivanyi, L. and Lehner, T. (1972). Cell mediated immunity in herpesvirus hominis infections. *Br. Med. J.*, **1**, 723–6

107. Shillitoe, E. J., Wilton, J. M. A. and Lehner, T. (1977). Sequential changes in cell-mediated immune responses to herpes simplex virus after recurrent herpetic infection in humans. *Infect. Immun.*, **18**, (1), 130–7

108. O'Reilly, R. J., Chibbaro, A., Anger, E. and Lopez, C. (1977). Cell-mediated immune responses in patients with recurrent herpes labialis or herpes progenitalis. *J. Immunol.*, **118** (3), 1095–102

109. Easty, D. L., Carter, C. and Funk, A. (1981). Systemic immunity in herpetic keratitis. *Br. J. Ophthalmol.*, **65**, 82–8

110. Ohno, S., Kato, F., Matsuda, H., Hosokawa, M. and Kobayashi, H. (1981). Delayed skin reactivity of patients with herpetic stromal keratitis. *Ann. Ophthalmol.*, **13**, 483–5

111. Hendricks, R. L. and Sugar, J. (1984). Lysis of herpes simplex virus infected targets. II Nature of the effector cell. *Cell. Immunol.*, **83**, 202–70

112. Dawson, C., Togni, B. and Moore, T. E. (1968). Structural changes in chronic herpetic keratitis. *Arch. Ophthalmol.*, **79**, 740–7

113. Meyers-Elliott, R. H., Pettit, T. H. and Maxwell, A. (1980). Viral antigens in the immune ring of herpes simplex stromal keratitis. *Arch. Ophthalmol.*, **98**, 897–904

114. Metcalf, J. F. and Kaufman, H. E. (1976). Herpetic stromal keratitis — evidence for cell-mediated immunopathogenesis. *Am. J. Ophthalmol.*, **82** (6), 827–34

115. Ahonen, R., Vannas, A. and Makitie, J. (1984). Virus particles and leukocytes in herpes simplex keratitis. *Cornea*, **3**, 43–50

116. Limberg, M. B., Margo, C. E. and Lyman, G. H. (1986). Eosinophils in corneas removed by penetrating keratoplasty. *Br. J. Ophthalmol.*, **70**, 343–6

117. Kanai, A. and Kaufman, H. E. (1982). The retrocorneal ridge in syphilitic and herpetic interstitial keratitis: an electron microscopic study. *Ann. Ophthalmol.*, **14**, 120–4

118. Youinou, P., Colin, J. and Ferec, C. (1986). Monoclonal antibody analysis of blood and cornea T lymphocyte subpopulations in herpes simplex keratitis. *Graefe's Arch. Clin. Exp. Ophthalmol.*, **224**, 131–3

119. Youinou, P., Colin, J. and Mottier, D. (1985). Immunological analysis of the cornea in herpetic stromal keratitis. *J. Clin. Lab. Immunol.*, **17**, 105–6

120. Jones, B. R., Falcon, M. G., Williams, H. P. and Coster, D. J. (1977). Symposium on Herpes Simplex Eye Disease: Objectives of Therapy of Herpetic Eye Disease. *Trans. Ophthalmol. Soc. U.K.*, **97**, 305–13

4
Immunology of Corneal Transplantation

M. G. FALCON

INTRODUCTION

There was considerable interest in corneal surgery, including grafting, in the early nineteenth century, but failure was universal because of a lack of understanding of immunology and corneal physiology. With improvements in asepsis and anaesthesia later in the same century, some progress was made, and the first successful human lamellar graft was performed in 1886 by von Hippel. The next 50 years saw further interest in the possibilities of corneal transplantation, and further (though rather crude) progress; but it was not until after the Second World War that most of the major advances were made, leading to a far greater chance of success. None of these advances has been more important than the development of immunology. Indeed, the cornea has been an excellent model for transplantation immunology in general. Following Maumenee's[1] recognition that clinical rejection can occur, and the experimental work of Khodadoust and Silverstein[2] that evaluated this in detail, we realize today that corneal graft rejection is the commonest cause of graft failure, and (now that most other difficulties have been largely overcome) it is by far the most taxing problem that remains.

This chapter is designed to cover the relevant background of transplantation immunology with particular reference to the cornea, and it examines the pathogenesis and clinical forms of rejection. The clinical management and pharmacological treatment of rejection are considered, and some selected areas are discussed where further advances seem promising.

Corneal structure and function relevant to transplantation

The cornea is, of course, very specialized and unusual in its anatomy and physiology, and this has an important bearing on transplantation. There are three principal layers (Figure 4.1). The *epithelium* is composed of stratified squamous non-keratinized cells about five layers thick, which are produced by the active basal cells at the limbal (corneoscleral) region. Within the epithelium are Langerhans cells, which are particularly concentrated at the

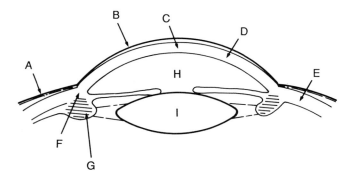

Figure 4.1 Schematic horizontal section of the eye. **A**. conjunctiva, with vessels; **B**, corneal epithelium; **C**, corneal stroma; **D**, corneal endothelium, and Descemet's membrane; **E**, sclera; **F**, drainage angle of anterior chamber; **G**, ciliary body; **H**, anterior chamber; **I**, lens

limbus, and they can also be found in vascular endothelium (corneal or other). The Langerhans cells are macrophage-derived antigen-presenting cells (APC), whose function is critical to transplantation immunology. Probably identical in function are the stromal interstitial dendritic cells, and the APC in the conjunctival epithelium associated with the localized lymphoid tissue in the conjunctival submucosa, known as CALT (conjunctiva-associated lymphoid tissue).

Beneath the epithelium there is a condensation of stroma termed Bowman's layer. The rest of the *stroma*, accounting for the most of the corneal thickness and strength, is composed of closely-packed and regularly-arranged lamellae of specialized collagen (which allows light transmission) embedded in a ground substance within which are keratocytes. The proteoglycans in the ground substance account for the considerable tendency of the stroma to swell osmotically. The stroma is devoid of lymphatics and blood vessels in health, but it can acquire them when diseased (corneal vascularization being a particularly common response to a variety of insults). Peripherally, the stroma joins the sclera at the limbus. It has a small component of interstitial dendritic cells. Other inflammatory cells such as polymorphs can move into and within the stroma (from the limbus or the aqueous humour), and this is greatly facilitated by certain pathological conditions.

On the internal limit of the stroma is Descemet's membrane, a tough, thin sheet of specialized collagen that is secreted by the endothelium throughout life. The *endothelium* (probably derived from neural crest) is a monolayer of epithelial cells that, in humans, normally have no capacity for mitosis. It has the critical function of pumping fluid out of the stroma into the anterior chamber, to maintain corneal transparency. If the endothelium fails, through (surgical) trauma, rejection or any other disease process, then corneal swelling will occur, and corneal transparency will be lost. Peripherally, the endothelium becomes involved, at the root of the iris, with the drainage mechanism that allows aqueous to leave the eye. This should normally balance aqueous production by the ciliary body and thus keep intraocular

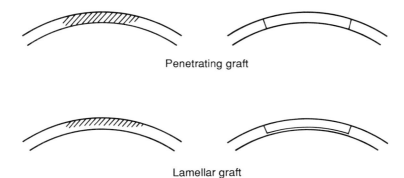

Penetrating graft

Lamellar graft

Figure 4.2 Types of corneal graft

pressure controlled. However, failure of aqueous drainage can occur for a variety of reasons, including states of inflammation, as can occur in corneal transplantation: raised intraocular pressure is an all too common complication that the ophthalmologist is always mindful of.

Types of corneal graft

For obvious reasons, the type of corneal transplant will be determined by the nature of the particular corneal disease, but there are two main groups of corneal graft: penetrating (PK) and lamellar. In a PK, the full thickness of cornea is replaced and the wound is secured with edge-to-edge sutures. These grafts are usually circular, and limited to the central 6–9 mm of cornea. If the endothelium is healthy, and if the corneal disease is confined to the anterior three-quarters (or less) of the stroma, it is possible to split the cornea horizontally, removing the diseased portion and replacing it with an appropriately cut donor piece — a lamellar graft. Provided it is reserved for appropriate patients, this has a number of important advantages, particularly immunological (Figure 4.2).

The donor

Once the donor eye has been removed, there are several methods of storage that have a bearing on transplantation.

Moist chamber storage enables the whole eye to be kept satisfactorily for about 24 hours before the cornea is used. A temperature of 4° C is obligatory: this slows down corneal (particularly endothelial) metabolism sufficiently to keep most of the cells alive, although they are obviously deprived of normal nutrients and exposed increasingly to metabolites. Beyond 24 hours, there is increasing endothelial disturbance and then death. The process is very simple, and reliable, and it has, until recently, been the most commonly used method of storage. It is rather less satisfactory (in view of the limited time available), now that donor HIV screening is obligatory, and also because more interest is being paid to tissue matching. Longer-term storage methods have been developed.

43

Medium-term corneal storage has been made feasible by the introduction of media that allow the endothelium to remain healthy for longer at 4°C. The two principal media concerned are either McCarey–Kaufman (MK) or chondroitin-sulphate-containing (KSol). With these, the corneoscleral disc can be stored safely for several days — probably up to 10 days in KSol and up to 3 in MK, although data vary considerably. As with the moist chamber method, corneal cells, particularly endothelium, should be preserved intact, but the impairment of endothelial function during storage leads to considerable corneal swelling; this reverses once the disc is in the recipient eye.

Organ-culture involves keeping the corneoscleral disc in a special and rather complex environment at 37°C, in which corneal metabolism is relatively normal. These corneas can be stored for up to 30 days, without significant impairment, and this allows leisurely evaluation of the tissue. More importantly, it increases the prospects that during this time a suitably matched recipient may be found. Perhaps most important of all is the observation that, after about 2 weeks, the epithelium becomes very thin, and loses its Langerhans cells. The same may be true of the stromal interstitial dendritic cells, and this gives rise to the possibility that organ-stored material may be less likely to initiate an allograft reaction. This is discussed later on.

CORNEAL TRANSPLANTATION: THE BACKGROUND

Although corneal disease in the Western world is relatively rare, the number of grafts performed in the UK seems to be increasing. This is probably due mainly to the fact that ophthalmologists now have higher expectations, and are prepared to take on patients for grafting who were previously left alone. Correspondingly, improvements in the results because of microsurgery, better availability of donor material and better postoperarative management all justify this enthusiasm. Some of these eyes, with complex problems, may eventually fail because of glaucoma or posterior segment disease; again, if the corneal environment is inappropriate, so perhaps was the graft in the first place. But outside these relatively particular problems it is the spectre of graft rejection that hovers over every patient, and it can even bring about long-term failure in those considered initially to be at low risk[3].

We need to define 'rejection': the term is sometimes misused to imply a failure of a graft for any reason where there is ultimately endothelial failure, when it should be used specifically to imply the immunological phenomena that can attack the graft. We thus use the term "(acute) rejection", which may (if successfully treated) or may not lead to permanent graft damage ("rejected graft") — one specific cause of a failed graft.

We need to look at the *fate of the transplanted material* to consider rejection in more detail. It is known that the epithelium is dynamic: if the grafted epithelium is removed (see page 54) the defect will be covered over by the host epithelium usually within a few days. If it is not removed the donor epithelium may persist for some weeks, or more rarely for longer. Experimentally, it can be rejected even after as long as 6 months. Clinically, the immunological destruction of epithelium is in itself unimportant because the deficit can be made up rapidly by the host.

The main cellular component of a stroma is the keratocytes, and these are rather indolent mitotically. Experimental studies again show that there is long-term keratocyte survival, and it has been shown by sex chromatin studies that some keratocytes from the donor may persist for up to 16 years. These probably represent the minority: most donor keratocytes have been replaced by host cells much earlier. The immunological destruction of donor keratocytes may thus be expected to produce clinical signs in the stroma, although there should be no long-lasting sequelae, as these cells can eventually be replaced with donor cells. This provides one of the major attractions of the lamellar graft.

As we have seen, the endothelium is critical to corneal deturgescence: every eye-bank worker and ophthalmologist knows that the quality of donor endothelium is of critical importance for the success of the penetrating graft. As the endothelium does not divide, the endothelial dose transplanted at surgery must last for the remainder of the patient's life. If it is inadequate right from the start, this constitutes primary graft failure; occasionally, it can be delayed for months or (more frequently) years — delayed graft failure. There is generally a considerable fall-out of graft endothelial counts during the 2 years after surgery, most probably because these cells need to move over to cover deficiencies in the host endothelium caused by the original disease or surgical trauma. Thereafter, graft endothelial counts are fairly stable, and delayed graft failure is surprisingly rare.

The long-term survival of grafted endothelium[4] is supported by experimental work, and by the clinical fact that endothelial rejection can occur after well over 10 years. The immunological destruction of grafted endothelium will provide obvious and immediate results that may also be manifest in the host tissue nearby if there has been significant donor endothelial cell movement. Not only will the functional effect be profound, but it may be irreversible if the endothelium is damaged beyond repair: *this is the central problem in corneal graft rejection.*

THE PRINCIPLES OF CORNEAL GRAFT IMMUNOLOGY

It was known by the late 1940s that damage to transplanted tissues occurred through immunological reactions[5], and that histocompatibility matching was required between donor and host for a successful transplant. The fact remained, however, that many unmatched corneal grafts were successful; this led to a number of concepts that were used to explain this phenomenon:

(1) *The cornea was not antigenic.* We now know that every nucleated cell in the body so far studied expresses the full range of host Class 1 HLA antigens. The antigenicity of corneal tissue was demonstrated long ago by experiments in which cornea was transplanted to vascular sites elsewhere in the body: it was readily rejected. Maumenee[1] subsequently showed that the cornea *in situ* could be involved in immunological rejection. There

followed the classical work of Khodadoust and Silverstein[2], who demonstrated experimentally that each of the three main corneal layers could initiate, and be involved in, the rejection process.

(2) The graft underwent some immunological change or adaptation that allowed it to be accepted by the host. The fact that rejection can occur up to many years after transplantation largely explodes this theory. There is rapid epithelial and gradual stromal cellular replacement by host tissue. From a theoretical point of view, any (immunological) process that led to long-term acceptance of a homograft would be of great value, and it may be in this direction that transplantation has a brighter future than it ever can with non-specific immunosuppression of the host.

(3) There was rapid death of grafted donor cells, with subsequent replacement by host. This may occur in the epithelium but, as discussed already, it is now well known that rapid replacement of dead keratocytes is not possible, and any replacement of dead endothelial cells is only possible by the gradual process of endothelial slide. Even if this were eventually to occur (and experience of primary graft failure indicates that it does not) there would be a prolonged period of severe endothelial decompensation first, which simply does not occur.

(4) Some particular features of the cornea, and in particular its avascularity, allowed the graft to remain sequestered from the host's immune system — the theory of 'corneal privilege'. Of the four concepts proposed, this is the only one to remain convincing, and there is now a good deal of experimental and clinical evidence to support it.

We shall consider later and in more detail the afferent (or sensitization) and the efferent (or destructive) phases of the rejection process. Both could be impeded by the particular structure of the cornea. Maumenee[6] demonstrated that host sensitization (sufficient to bring about subsequent rejection of the corneal graft) need not be induced from grafted corneal tissue, but did occur from grafted skin. This phenomenon is not absolute, however, since some patients with avascular grafts sometimes undergo graft rejection. Later workers have further shown that the mechanism can be broken down if the corneal graft is placed peripherally[7], or in an area of induced corneal vascularization, and we shall see later how this is relevant clinically.

Once a graft is established quietly in place, it is very likely to have a degree of protection from the host's immune system. This can probably occur even in a vascular cornea, if the blood/corneal barrier remains intact. A small disturbance, such as a loose suture, may be enough to neutralize this effect and allow the efferent phase to occur. It is worth bearing in mind, though, that the amount of 'tissue contact' (host to donor) is relatively much greater in a corneal graft than in, say, a renal graft, where, apart from the vascular and other anastomoses, there is none, but the blood–organ barrier is all the more important.

The importance of avascularity in the efferent limb was demonstrated first in 1953[8], and the experiments of Khodadoust and Silverstein[9] showed further that all vascular grafts were rejected following sensitization of the host at another site, whereas 25% of avascular grafts survived. Finally, it should be borne in mind that there are alternative pathways for the rejection mechanism other than blood vessels: cells can migrate from the iris to the cornea via the aqueous, or they can cross the cornea from the limbus.

We now need to look at the pathogenesis of corneal graft rejection, and this brings us first to consider the basic immunology of transplantation.

Transplantation immunology

How is it that individuality is expressed at a cellular level; and how are the genetic differences between individuals of the same (vertebrate) species, as well as between different species, recognized immunologically (and, if appropriate, used to bring about a graft rejection)?

The mechanism that labels nucleated cells with an individual's identity is a closely linked cluster of genes (on chromosome 6 in man), termed the major histocompatibility complex (MHC), and known as the human leukocyte antigen (HLA) system in man. The HLA system was originally identified by its ability to provoke rejection[10], but its natural role is more concerned with the individual's ability to distinguish between self and non-self (which may mimic self) in the fight against external agents, particularly through infection.

The HLA genes are a linked complex of at least three gene families that give rise to three classes of antigens. Class I antigens are encoded by the HLA A, HLA B and HLA C regions; Class II antigens are from the HLA D region, which can be subdivided into HLA DP, HLA DQ and HLA DR regions; and Class III antigens are involved with complement components and two different 21-hydroxylase enzymes; they are not involved in the rejection process.

Class I antigens are glycoproteins found on the surface of all nucleated cells (except for villous trophoblast). T cells of the killer subset (CD8+) do not recognize free antigen but need to see it in the context of self Class I antigens on the surface of the antigen-presenting cells (APC). The combined complex of antigen and Class I antigens interact with the CD8+ T-cell receptor. Other CD8+ T cells recognize foreign Class I antigens on the cell surface. Both types of interaction can result in cytolysis and death of the target cell bearing the Class I antigens; this most commonly involves destruction of cells containing virus antigen in the former case, and destruction of allograft cells in the latter.

The Class II HLA antigens are also glycoproteins. They are normally restricted to B cells and macrophages, and other cells involved directly with the immune response[11]. They can sometimes be aberrantly expressed on non-lymphoid cells, too, such as epithelium and endothelium, when these tissues are exposed to lymphokines such as interferon gamma[12]. Class II antigens serve as restriction elements for T-helper (CD4+) cells. These cells interact with antigen together with self Class II antigens on the surface of APC via the T-cell receptor, and are then activated. Foreign Class II antigens on the cell surface can also be recognized by some CD4+ T cells. CD4+ T cells have a variety of functions in that they can secrete interleukin-2, allowing

47

maturation of CD8+ cytotoxic T cells and helper B cells. They may also have a primary effector role in that some subtypes of CD4+ cells (Th1) are able to kill target cells expressing antigen plus Class II antigens.

It thus appears that both CD8+ T cells (directed at Class I antigens) and CD4+ T cells (stimulated by Class II antigens) are involved in MHC incompatibility reactions and the exact cell type involved will depend on the HLA antigens expressed[13].

The pathogeneis of corneal graft rejection

The afferent limb

This section considers the processes that lead to recognition by the host that foreign material is in the cornea. Central to this are the Langerhans[14,15] and similar APC, and it is now appreciated that donor-derived APC are of greater importance in initiating rejection than those in the host: they are a strong antigenic stimulus, bearing Class II antigens on their surface, and therefore interact directly with host CD4+ cells. The immunogenicity of different allograft tissues (bone marrow highest, liver lower and cornea lowest) can be related to the number of Class II bearing cells within them. Only very few donor APC are needed for this process, and various schemes have been tried to reduce their numbers. The fact that smaller grafts are rarely rejected could be seen as a result of the small number of APC introduced, but other factors are also involved. More importantly, experimental and even clinical depletion of donor APC, as with hyperbaric oxygen or ultraviolet light, has shown some encouraging results[16], and the use of organ-stored material (which loses its Langerhans cells after 2 weeks) may prove beneficial. So, too, should removal of the epithelium. A further important discovery is that both corneal epithelial and endothelial cells can be induced to express Class II antigens by lymphokines such as interferon gamma, which may be released by activated T cells in conditions such as uveitis. This could produce a self-perpetuating cycle once graft rejection has begun; it may also explain why rejection may appear to be triggered by other inflammatory episodes, such as recurrent herpetic disease, within the eye. There are, of course, other factors that can contribute, such as breakdown of the blood/aqueous barrier, allowing an influx of immunocompetent cells.

Elimination of the most powerful antigenic determinants in the graft would obviously be the ideal way to tackle the rejection problem, and it contrasts dramatically with the wanton anti-inflammatory and immunosuppressive treatment that we use at present. Tissue matching is a satisfactory theoretical alternative (discussed later), but there will always be poor prospects for a really good match for numerical and logistical reasons.

In the absence of Class II antigens on the donor cells, the afferent limb must occur through recipient Langerhans cells, which must process the donor Class I antigens before the cytoxic CD8+ cells can be stimulated. This response is much weaker — the chance of rejection is thus considerably less than for Class II antigens. Nevertheless, we have seen that Class I antigens are expessed throughout the corneal cells, and Class I matching has been shown to be of some benefit.

At the other end of the interaction, a relationship has been shown between the incidence of graft rejection and the Langerhans cell count in the excised disc[15] (presumably reflecting the count in the remaining host tissue). This gives another justification for pretreatment with steroids in patients whose grafts are performed when the eye is inflamed; and it is but one demonstration of the situation, probably unique to the eye, in which the *recipient* state is important in determining the incidence of rejection.

The efferent limb

Following activation of CD4+ T cells, various coordinated events, including the release of interleukin-2, lead to the production of CD8+ cells from cytotoxic T-cell precursors. These are specifically directed against cells bearing foreign Class I antigens. Whether CD4+ cells have an effector role as well is not clear.

There is uncertainty about the precise location of these events: any aggregation of lymphoid tissue will probably suffice, particularly if adjacent to the eye; thus the limbus, the CALT[17], and local lymph nodes are probably involved more than the spleen and more distant lymphoid tissue.

The route for the efferent limb is principally vascular, although this is not essential, since grafts in avascular corneas can reject; there may be direct migration of cells into the cornea from the limbus, from the iris (direct to the cornea if there are anterior synechiae), or via the aqueous, but the blood–aqueous barrier limits access to the cornea.

Pathology

Pathologically, the features of rejection are much as would be expected from our understanding of the pathogenesis[18,19]: there is a focal infiltration with lymphocytes and a few polymorphs in the tissue undergoing rejection (whether epithelial or endothelial) and there is corresponding focal damage to these tissues. The affected epithelium is readily replaced with normal (host) epithelium, but the affected endothelium is replaced eventually by a sheet of fibroblast-like cells, leading to the 'retro-graft membrane'. This may be derived from metaplasia of the affected endothelial cells or from fibroblasts coming from the graft host junction.

In the stroma, where rejection is much less common, the changes may be confused by those derived from endothelial rejection (stromal oedema and infiltration, and ultimately vascularization). However, true stromal rejection has been produced experimentally; it shows infiltration with lymphocytes and plasma cells, and later fibroblasts; these lead to destruction of the epithelial basement membrane and severe abnormalities in the keratocytes that can likewise be destroyed, with consequent destruction of local collagen synthesis.

The role of antibody in corneal graft rejection

Although antibody may play an important part in rejection of vascular allografts, this does not appear to be the case with the cornea. Anticorneal antibodies can be demonstrated after grafting, both experimentally and clinically, and there may be a sustained high titre in failing grafts, but it is not clear whether these have developed in relation to (surgical) trauma or more specifically to grafting[20]. Early work found an apparent association between antibodies in the host and unresponsive graft rejection, and if these were present before surgery, the prognosis was correspondingly worse[21].

These humoral mechanisms may play a central role in some corneal diseases such as Mooren's ulcer, and it is striking, and very fortunate, that such peripheral corneal destruction in never a feature of graft rejection.

CLINICAL FEATURES OF CORNEAL GRAFT REJECTION

Our examination of the pathogenesis of graft rejection makes interpretation of the clinical features very straightforward; indeed, there can be no other area where immunopathology can be so directly viewed.

Accelerated graft rejection

We have noted that primary graft failure leads, for obvious reasons, to a decompensated graft right from the first postoperative day. A partly or completely decompensated graft within the first 10 postoperative days, in association with active uveitis and KP on the graft endothelium, is almost certainly caused by a so-called 'accelerated graft rejection', although there may occasionally be doubts as, for instance, when the corneal surgery has been combined with cataract or vitreous surgery, that could perhaps be to blame. An accelerated graft reaction is now extremely rare. It is caused by sensitization of the host to HLA antigens by a previous donor. When this HLA antigen is present on the new graft, an explosive immune reaction occurs and this results in very rapid rejection of that graft (second set phenomenon). This disastrous development is usually very florid, and rarely responds to treatment. There is the hope, naturally, that a subsequent graft may not contain any of the relevant antigens.

Classical allograft rejection

The timing of rejection is of great importance to the clinician. Not only is it impossible for a rejection episode (except an accelerated graft rejection) to occur in less than 10 days of grafting for immunological reasons, but it is also very rarely that rejection occurs within a few months. This is most probably because of the intensity of the topical steroid treatment early on, and it makes the important point that rejection could usually be prevented if sufficient steroid were continued for long enough. However, the clinician has no means of determining how long this is, and balanced against this are the very real dangers, particularly of raised intraocular pressure and cataract, that accompany prolonged topical steroid therapy. Sometimes added to this are particular factors, such as herpetic keratitis, that further turn one away from prolonged steroids. Yet it is worthy of note that it is the risk (and hence, from the point of view of the graft, the inadequate use) of steroid that could be blamed for most episodes of rejection: they rarely occur when the steroid

50

treatment is in full swing. Thus, the peak time for classical allograft rejection is between about 4 and 18 months postoperatively, thereafter declining steadily. After 5 years, rejection is very rare, but it has been known even after more than 10 years.

Epithelial rejection

Although donor epithelium may be deliberately removed by the surgeon, or it may be very attenuated in organ stored corneoscleral discs, there are still circumstances in which it is transplanted more or less intact. Thoft[22], moreover, has advocated transplantation of donor epithelium (where the fellow eye cannot provide adequate epithelium) to deal with the severe surfacing problems in alkali burns ('keratoepithelioplasty'). Under the influence of postoperative steroids, epithelium can persist for weeks or months, and an epithelial rejection line may be seen during this time. The appearances are of an irregular line of haze and infiltration at almost any site in the donor epithelium — appearances superficially resembling herpetic or mucous plaque keratitis. Because the immunologically-destroyed epithelium is replaced rapidly by host tissue, there are obviously no long-lasting sequelae. It is, however, uncomfortable to realize that the occurrence of epithelial rejection means that the host is already sensitized against donor antigens, indicating that there is a risk of endothelial (and stromal) rejection: the afferent limb has already occurred.

Stromal rejection

Stromal rejection seems to be rare. This observation could be erroneous, because the clinical signs are minor, or misinterpreted, but a low incidence of stromal rejection would be expected because the stroma is far less cellular than epithelium or endothelium. Clinical signs that have been attributed to it are focal nummular opacities or subepithelial infiltrates, first described by Krachmer and Allredge in 1978[23]. They reported an incidence of 15%, but the incidence may vary greatly with the masking effect of topical steroids: the lesions fade (or are suppressed) readily with such treatment. The opacities resemble those of adenovirus keratoconjunctivitis.

Though scarring could ensue if there were actual destruction of collagen, and destruction of keratocytes could delay the process of repair, the results of stromal rejection are far less serious than those of endothelial rejection for obvious physiological reasons. Stromal rejection may often be accompanied by endothelial rejection and its clinical signs may therefore be masked by it.

Endothelial rejection

This is so central to corneal graft rejection that the term 'rejection' is often used for it. There are usually some symptoms accompanying the clinical signs: redness, discomfort or pain, photophobia and blurred vision.

The clinical signs are a vivid demonstration of applied immunology and corneal pathophysiology (Figure 4.3). Typically, there is a localized area

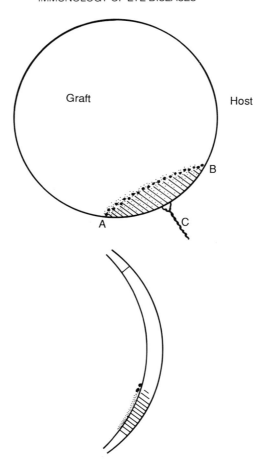

Figure 4.3 Classical endothelial rejection (A/P and vertical section). A–B Khodadoust line; C, corneal blood vessel. Cross-hatching indicates area of endothelial damage and consequent stromal swelling

towards the periphery of the graft of stromal and perhaps epithelial oedema (representing the endothelial damage), where the endothelium shows an accumulation of KP, typically in a line concentric with the graft/host junction (Khodadoust's line), and there are cells in the anterior chamber. There may be an adjacent host vessel, or anterior synechia, that provides the route of the efferent limb (it may have been the route for the afferent limb, too). The KP are of course composed of aggregations of CD8+ T cells and probably some CD4+ T cells, and will moved forwards (centrally) destroying endothelial cells as they go. Though some of the endothelial disturbance may be reversible, it is clearly a matter of urgency that treatment be started straight away.

Endothelial rejection is sometimes diffuse (Figure 4.4); here the T cells come (from the iris) through the aqueous, and attack the entire graft

Host

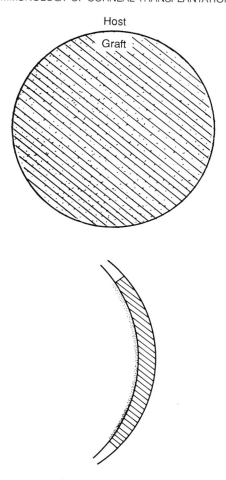

Figure 4.4 Diffuse endothelial rejection (A/P and vertical section). Cross-hatching indicates area of endothelial damage and consequent stromal swelling

endothelium. The appearances can be identical to the disciform keratitis of herpes simplex. Since some grafts are carried out for hereptic keratitis, this can pose a difficult clinical dilemma. Only when the KP and associated endothelial decompensation extend well beyond the graft can one confidently implicate the virus rather than rejection. The importance is that in the latter, the graft has a better prognosis, and relatively little steroid (with antiviral cover) is required, whereas in a rejection, intensive steroids are essential, no matter what the reason for the graft.

RISK FACTORS FOR CORNEAL GRAFT REJECTION

A great deal of clinical study has been directed towards identifying prognostic indicators in corneal graft rejection[24,25] because the difference in outcome between a successful graft and a rejected one is so profound: it may mean the difference between normal vision and less vision than preoperatively. Many of the risk factors are quite consistent with the expectations following from our study of graft rejection.

Donor factors

Several factors in the host tissue may influence the incidence of rejection. As discussed already, the central issue is the number of Langerhans cells (and interstitial dendritic cells).

The Langerhans cell count will be greater in larger grafts, and this may be of some relevance (along with host factors discussed shortly) in influencing the rejection rate. It has also been noticed that renal grafts from donors who were immunosuppressed at the time of death have a rather lower chance of being rejected — perhaps for similar reasons.

One of the most important debates in corneal grafting has concerned removal of the donor epithelium. As indicated earlier, the epithelial cells are a strong source of class I HLA antigens (as well as containing Langerhans cells) and it should make good clinical sense, therefore, to remove the donor epithelium at the time of surgery in order to reduce the antigenic load. Until very recently, however, there has been no clear evidence that this does make a difference. Several studies have attempted to resolve the issue, with conflicting results, but careful analysis of these reports raises some uncertainties that may explain why there was no overall agreement. Stulting et al.[26] have now shown, in a randomized prospective study of 332 keratoplasties, that removal of donor epithelium did not reduce the incidence of graft failure, irreversible allograft rejection or reversible allograft rejection. The technique of epithelial removal was shown histologically to be satisfactory. This study used short-term storage (up to 4 days), which is unlikely to affect donor antigenicity. The randomization was stratified so that patients who were at high risk of rejection were equally distributed between the two groups, and the mean follow-up time was two years.

There was a persistent trend in favour of the eye that had the epithelium left *on* when considering definite rejection; definite and probable rejection; and definite, probable, and possible rejection. The greatest difference (approaching statistical significance) was when all causes of graft failure were considered together: those whose donor epithelium was left in place at the time of surgery seemed to do better.

This important and well-planned study seems finally to denounce any benefit from donor epithelial removal in reducing graft rejection — a rather surprising result in view of the logic.

Host factors

Graft size is important. Very small grafts have several non-immunological drawbacks, and are rarely performed these days. Large grafts, beyond 7.5–8.00 mm, have a higher incidence of rejection[27], probably because they are likely to extend towards vascular tissue or towards the limbus in the host, and possibly also because they represent a larger antigenic load, as discussed already.

Graft position is also relevant For very similar reasons, central grafts do better than peripherally placed ones, where the incidence of rejection is significantly higher[28,29].

Recipient age has a slight bearing on graft rejection: the incidence is less in older recipients, presumably because of an overall decline in the activity of the immune system.

Anterior synechiae to the graft/host junction are a risk factor for rejection, because of the vascularity of the iris[30]: though these should be rare nowadays with modern surgical techniques, it has been not uncommon in the past to see an endothelial rejection line arising at the site of such synechiae.

Vascularization is profoundly important, and the incidence of rejection has been shown to be linked to the degree of vascularization (in quadrants) in several studies[3,30–33]. It is still not clear whether the vessels alone are sufficient to encourage rejection, or whether it is the presence of lymphatics, which can accompany corneal blood vessels. The influence of vascularization is highly significant, and all corneal surgeons rightly tend to shy away from grafting in such situations, unless matching is possible.

Grafting an inflamed eye ('à chaud') has been well shown to increase the chance of subsequent rejection, as have the following:

- *A background of inflammatory eye disease* such as may be associated with keratoconus, or herpetic keratitis, may increase the likelihood of rejection for obvious reasons.

- *Previous grafts* are a risk factor. Rejection being the commonest form of failure, this means that there could be pre-existing sensitization to one or more of the antigens in the new donor[1,30,33]. The chance for this is in fact remarkably low, and it has been argued that it is repeated surgery and its consequences (vascularization, synechiae, and perhaps larger subsequent grafts) that really affect the likelihood of rejection.

- *Pre-treatment of the host with steroids* is likely to decrease the influence of some of these factors, by reducing vascularization, reducing Langerhans cell counts in the host periphery and limbus[15], and generally depressing many aspects of the immune process. Though there is so little data to prove its value, it is probably employed all too rarely.

- *Postoperative influences* can be profoundly important. So often a graft rejection is triggered by vascularization or inflammation from a loose suture, or recurrence of inflammatory disease (herpes simplex); or merely from premature reduction in preventive topical steroid therapy either by an ill-informed surgeon or by a misinformed patient.

Though many of these factors have a profound influence of the incidence of graft rejection, many of them may be unavoidable in the clinical context. A great deal of work has correspondingly been directed to avoidable factors, and by far the most researched of these has been the issue of tissue matching.

Tissue matching

There are around 20 known alleles on the HLA-A locus, 35 on the B locus, 10 on the C, and 10 on the D. This obviously leads to a huge number of combinations with a very remote chance that two individuals could be matched completely. However, some degree of matching can be beneficial, and the tissue typing process is still based on the work of Terasaki and McClelland (1964)[34].

HLA antigens can induce an antibody response, which has been implicated in the rapid failure of vascular transplants. Such patients are now routinely tested preoperatively to ensure that they have not previously been sensitized to the potential donor's antigens. It is not clear whether the mechanism can have a role in corneal graft failure: evidence is so far to the contrary.

Blood group antigens

Although blood group antigens A, B and O are present in the corneal epithelium, this probably has minimal relevance to the outcome of corneal grafting. In vascular transplants, particularly the kidney, the situation is very different.

The value of HLA matching has been extensively investigated in a number of corneal transplantation centres — in Europe notably at East Grinstead in England[24,33], and at Leyden in the Netherlands[35]. It has been shown clearly and with reasonable consistency that patients who are at high risk of rejection, particularly because of corneal vascularization, do benefit significantly with the use of reasonably matched tissue, whereas it is hard to show a benefit in the low-risk patients (rejection being so uncommon anyway). These factors are not disputed, and it is probably true to say that, were there not financial and logistical limitations[36], matching would be welcomed with much more enthusiasm by all corneal surgeons. It is a great pity that, so far, rather little corneal material has been available from renal and heart donors (who have often already been tissue typed); progress is being made through the national and international transplant services such as UKTS and Eurotransplant.

The work of the East Grinstead group led by Casey[24,33] exemplifies the progress that has been made towards identifying the value of matching. In 450 grafts reviewed over 14 years, patients were divided into low-, medium- and high-risk groups. The first group of 142 grafts contained first grafts in avascular corneas; in the second group (156 grafts) were patients with up to two quadrants of vascularization and up to two previous grafts; those in the high-risk group (152) had more than two quadrants of vascularization and more than two previously rejected grafts. Patients in the low-risk group did very well regardless of the quality of tissue matching: at 2 years postoperatively, 88% of those with no antigens matched had clear grafts; 94% of those with one antigen matched were clear; 90% were clear for two matches, and

100% for three antigen matches. Thus, there seemed, in this extensive series, to be a slight benefit from matching even in these low-risk patients, but the view of many corneal surgeons continues to be that the slight (though, theoretically, definite) benefit afforded does not justify the very considerable expenditure of resources. In the medium-risk group, the corresponding figures for clear grafts were 76%, 78%, 90% and 100% at 2 years for the four degrees of matching. This achieves significance at the $P<0.1$ level if the first and second groups are compared with the second and third (76% clear graft rate versus 92%).

For the high-risk group, the figures are 57%, 51%, 74% and 69% (rather less at 1 year); significance at the $P<0.1$ level is achieved with similar grouping as for the medium-risk group: 50% of the no-match or single-match grafts were clear compared with 76% of the grafts with two or three matches.

Similar results have come from the Leyden[35] group and from the United States[37]. Perhaps even more interesting is the value of Class II matching (so far demonstrated in renal transplantation) that should prove, in the light of current knowledge, more central to reducing corneal rejection than matching Class I antigens. A small series from Leyden indicated that Class II mismatching (at DRw6) gave a worse prognosis[38], and a study from Canada[39] showed that DR matching was of benefit. Prospective studies are under way in several centres.

TREATMENT OF CORNEAL GRAFT REJECTION

Once rejection has begun, a clear strategy of management is required: prompt and proper treatment will lead to resolution of the rejection, and the damage done by it, in the majority of patients.

Topical steroids

An initial subconjunctival injection of betamethasone (4 mg) or equivalent provides a satisfactory initial steroid load, and a strong mydriatic/cycloplegic (either atropine or hyoscine) should be given at the same time. This reduces any discomfort produced by the rejection episode, and also impedes the escape of protein and cells from the iris. Intensive topical steroids should be started soon, and continued with vigour at night (or replaced by ointment). There are usually visible signs of waning inflammation within a few days, although endothelial function may take weeks or even months to recover. The steroid therapy can thus be reduced gradually, but this needs to be done with caution: it may be best to continue with a 'preventive' load of topical steroid for many months after the rejection episode, in order to avoid recurrence. This has to be balanced against the risks.

Systemic steroids

The role of systemic steroids role remains uncertain. There are valid reasons for giving them — particularly the aim of reducing the production of CD8+

cells at sites distant from the eye. Nevertheless, the effect of topical steroid is so strong that one doubts whether any distant effect from systemic steroids would be of any extra value.

Cyclosporin A

Cyclosporin A is small cyclic polypeptide produced by a fungus and has a specific immunosuppressive effect by inhibiting the production of interleukin by activated T cells. It has found a valuable role in the transplantation of vascular organs[40] (kidney, liver, heart), although toxicity, particularly renal, must be constantly watched for, particularly by blood levels. There has been limited systemic use in corneal transplantation for this very reason, although experimental work has shown a beneficial effect, which did not persist for very long after the drug was stopped[7,41]. There were also demonstrations of a beneficial effect from topical therapy, either retrobulbar or subconjunctival, or as drops. Cyclosporin A is an oily liquid and it presents problems for delivery to the eye. Overall, it looks rather as though cyclosporin A will find only a minor role in corneal transplantation because of its toxicity[42]; topical steroids are very effective therapy, and further progress is probably to be made more at specific immunological sites rather than in generalized immunosuppression.

FUTURE PROSPECTS

There are several areas that offer prospects for improving the prognosis in corneal transplantation. From the immunological point of view, it is worth considering measures aimed at reducing antigenicity; possible methods for using the patients' own tissues; and means of producing more highly specific immunosuppression.

Reducing antigenicity

The importance of Langerhans cells, and possible means of reducing their numbers, have been discussed already. Reducing or masking donor antigens from the recipient is an additional possibility that has been investigated experimentally[43,44]. The aim would be that blocking antibody could be used to cover the donor antigen sites, thus eliminating or reducing rejection. The results have been variable so far, but obviously this possibility is highly attractive.

Autogenous tissue

Another approach would be to use the patient's own cells, or tissue, and some progress has been made in this respect. Epidermal growth factor has recently been shown to induce mitosis in the human endothelium[45], and this obviously has great clinical potential. An alternative possibility is the use of a patient's vascular endothelium (always readily available), with its capacity for mitosis;

58

would this behave appropriately like corneal endothelium when on Descemet's membrane? If either of these possibilities could lead to grafting the patient's own endothelium (even on to the stroma of an allograft), all the serious problems of rejection would eliminated, since stromal and epithelial rejection have minimal functional significance.

More specific immunosuppression

In the cornea, this would only be considered a feasible advance if it were applicable topically (viz., the unsuitability of systemic cyclosporin A in corneal patients).

References

These are but a representative selection of the large number of recent publications concerned with corneal graft immunology.

1. Maumenee, A. E. (1955). The immune concept: its relation to corneal homotransplantation. *Ann. N.Y. Acad. Sci.*, **59**, 453
2. Khodadoust, A. A. and Silverstein, A. M. (1969). Transplantation and rejection of individual cell layers of the corneal. *Invest. Ophthalmol.*, **8**, 180
3. Khodadoust, A. A. (1973). The allograft rejection reaction: the leading cause of late failure of clinical corneal grafts. In Jones, B. R. (ed.) *Corneal Graft Failure*. Ciba Foundation Symposium No. 15. (Amsterdam: Elsevier)
4. Chi, H. H., Teng, C. C. and Katzen, H. M. (1965). The fate of endothelial cells in corneal homografts. *Am. J. Ophthalmol.*, **59**, 186
5. Medawar, P. (1948). Immunity to homologous grafted skin. II. The fate of skin homografts transplanted to the brain, to subcutaneous tissue and anterior chamber of eye. *Br. J. Exp. Pathol.*, **29**, 58
6. Maumenee, A. E. (1951). The influence of donor recipient sensitisation on corneal grafts. *Am. J. Ophthalmol.*, **34**, 142
7. Hunter, P. A., Rice, N. S. C. and Jones, B. R. (1982). Prolonged corneal graft survival using topically applied cyclosporin A. *Trans. Ophthalmol. Soc. U.K.*, **1**, 19
8. Billingham, R. E. and Boswell, T. (1953). Studies on the problem of corneal homografts. *Proc. R. Soc. Lond. B*, **141**, 392
9. Khodadoust, A. A. and Silverstein, A. M. (1972). Studies on the nature of the privilege enjoyed by corneal allografts. *Invest. Ophthalmol.*, **11**, 137
10. Batchelor, J. R. (1975). Identification of HL-A antigens by serological criteria. *Ann. Rheum. Dis.*, **34** (Suppl. 1), 4
11. Hammerling, G. (1976). Tissue distribution of Ia (II) antigens and their expression on lymphocyte subpopulations. *Transplant. Rev.*, **30**, 64
12. Winman, K., Cunman, B., Forsum, V. *et al.* (1978). Occurrence of Ia (II) antigen on tissue of non-lymphoid origin. *Nature*, **276**, 711
13. Loveland, B. E. and McKenzie, I. F. C. (1982). Which T cells cause graft rejection? *Transplantation*, **33**, 2
14. Gillette, T. E., Chandler, J. W. and Greiner, J. V. (1982). Langerhans cells of the ocular surface. *Ophthalmology*, **89**, 700
15. Williams, K. A. and Coster, D. J. (1989). The role of the limbus in corneal allograft rejection. *Eye*, **3**, 158.
16. Ray-Keil, L., Gillette, T. E. and Chandler, J. W. (1985). Murine heterotopic corneal transplantation: reduction in rejection rates by pretreatment of donor corneas with ultraviolet light. *Invest. Ophthalmol., Vis. Sci.*, **26** (3, suppl.), 78
17. Chandler, J. W. and Axelrod, A. J. (1980). Conjunctiva-associated lymphoid tissue. In O'Connor, G. R. (ed.) *Immunologic Disease of Mucous Membranes*, (New York: Masson)
18. Polack, F. M. (1972). Scanning electron microscopy of corneal graft rejection: Epithelial rejection, endothelial rejection and formation of posterior graft membranes. *Invest.*

59

Ophthalmol., **11**, 1

19. Polack, F. M. (1973). Clinical and pathological aspects of the corneal graft reaction. *Trans. Am. Acad. Ophthalmol. Otolaryngol.*, **77**, 418

20. Grunnett, N., Kristensen, T. and Kissmeyer-Nielsen, F. (1976). Occurrence of lymphocytoxic lymphocytes and antibodies after corneal transplantation. *Acta. Ophthalmol.*, **54**, 167

21. Stark, W. J., Opelz, G., Newsome, D. *et al.* (1978). Sensitization to human lymphocyte antigens by corneal transplantation. *Invest. Ophthalmol.*, **12**, 639

22. Thoft, R. A. (1984). Keratoepithelioplasty. *Am. J. Ophthalmol.*, **97**, 1

23. Krachmer, J. H. and Alldredge, O. C. (1978). Subepithelial infiltrates: a probable sign of corneal transplant rejection. *Arch. Ophthalmol.*, **96**, 2234

24. Casey, T. A. and Mayer, D. J. (1984). *Corneal Grafting* (San Francisco: W. B. Saunders)

25. Coster, D. J. (1981). Factors affecting the outcome of corneal transplantation. *Ann. R. Coll. Surg. Engl.*, **63**, 91

26. Stulting, R. D., Waring, G. O., Bridges, W. Z. and Cavanagh, H. D. (1988). Effect of donor epithelium on corneal transplant survival. *Ophthalmology*, **95**, 803

27. Volker-Dieben, H. J., D'Amais, J. and Kok-van Alphen, C. C. (1987). Hierarchy of prognostic factors for corneal allograft survival. *Aust. N.Z. J. Ophthalmol.*, **15**, 11

28. Khodadoust, A. A. and Silverstein, A. M. (1972). Studies on the nature of the privilege enjoyed by corneal allografts. *Invest. Ophthalmol.*, **11**, 137

29. Wessels, I. F. and Dahan, E. (1986). Eccentric corneal grafts. *Am. J. Ophthalmol.*, **101**, 113

30. Arentsen, J. J. (1983). Corneal transplant allograft reaction: possible predisposing factors. *Trans. Am. Ophthalmol. Soc.*, **81**, 361

31. Alldredge, O. C. and Krachmer, J. H. (1981). Clinical types of corneal rejection: their manifestations, frequency, preoperative correlates, and treatment. *Arch. Ophthalmol.*, **99**, 599

32. Cherry, P. M. H. *et al.* (1979). An analysis of corneal transplantation: I. Graft clarity. *Ann. Ophthalmol.*, **II**, 461

33. Batchelor, J. R., Casey, T. A., West, A., Gibbs, D. C., Prasad, S. S., Lloyd, D. F. and James, A. (1976). HLA matching and corneal grafting. *Lancet*, **1**, 551

34. Terasaki, P. I. and McClelland, J. D. (1984). Microdroplet assay of human serum cytotoxins. *Nature*, **204**, 998

35. Volker-Dieben, H. J., Kok van Alphen, C. C. and Krut, P. J. (1979). Advances and disappointments, indications and restrictions regarding HLA matched corneal grafts in high risk cases. *Doc. Ophthalmol.*, **46**, 219

36. Watson, P. G. and Joysey, V. C. (1973). Difficulties in the use of tissue typing for corneal grafting. In Jones, B. R. (ed.) *Corneal Graft Failure*. Ciba Foundation Symposium, No. 15, p. 323. (Amsterdam: Elsevier)

37. Sanfilippo, F., MacQueen, J. M., Vaughn, W. K. and Foulks, G. N. (1986). Reduced graft rejection with good HLA-A matching in high-risk corneal transplantation. *N. Engl. J. Med.*, **315**, 29–35

38. Kok Van Alphen, C. C. (1982). The effect of prospective HLA-A and B matching on corneal graft survival. Presented to the International Cornea Society. Las Vegas, 1982

39. Boisjoly, H. M., Roy, R., Dubé, I., Laughrea, P. A., Michand, R., Douville, P. and Hébat, J. (1986). HLA-A, B and DR matching in corneal transplantation. *Ophthalmology*, **93**, 1290

40. Calne, R. Y. (1979). Immunosuppression for organ grafting: observations on cyclosporin A. *Immunol. Rev.*, **46**, 113

41. Coster, D. J., Shepherd, W. F., Fook, T. C. *et al.* (1979). Prolonged survival of corneal allografts in rabbits treated with cyclosporin A. Letter, *Lancet* **2**, 688

42. Hoffmann, F. and Widerbolt, M. (1986). Topical cyclosporin A in the treatment of corneal graft rejection. (Editorial) *Cornea* **5**, 129

43. Binder, P. S., Gebhardt, B. M. and Chandler, J. W. (1975). Immunologic protection of rabbit corneal allografts with heterologous blocking antibody. *Am. J. Ophthalmol.*, **79**, 949

44. Chandler, J. W., Gebhardt, B. M., Sugar, J. and Kaufman, H. E. (1973). Immunologic protection of corneal allografts: survival of cornea pretreated with heterologous "blocking" antibody. *Transplantation* **17**, 147

45. Couch, J. M., Cullen, P., Casey, T. A. and Fabre, J. W. (1987). Mitotic activity of corneal endothelial cells in organ culture with recombinant human epidermal growth factor. *Ophthalmology*, **94**, 1

5
Basic Mechanisms in Immune-mediated Uveitic Disease

R. R. CASPI

In order to study the immunopathogenic mechanisms that might underlie immune-mediated uveitic diseases in the human, it is necessary to employ experimental models of uveitis in laboratory animals. The best-studied immunologically mediated ocular inflammation is experimental autoimmune uveoretinitis (EAU), of which several models have been developed and are continuing to be developed in various rodent species as well as in primates. EAU serves as a model for a variety of posterior uveitic conditions in man, among them sympathetic ophthalmia, birdshot retinochoroidopathy, Behçet's disease and Vogt–Koyanagi–Harada (VKH) syndrome. All animal EAU models employ immunization of a susceptible animal species with one of several antigens extracted from the retina, injected as emulsion in complete Freund's adjuvant (CFA), at a site distant from the target organ. Immune lymphocytes then find their way to the target organ and induce the histopathological lesions typical of EAU. EAU is characterized by destruction of the photoreceptor cells of the retina, where the eliciting antigen(s) is located, and is usually accompanied by autoimmune inflammation of the pineal gland ("third eye") which shares many ocular-specific antigens with the retina. Although the fine details of EAU pathology and clinical manifestations vary from species to species, EAU can be classified as primarily a posterior segment inflammation, developing into a panuveitis in its more acute forms. Lesions such as photoreceptor damage, serous retinal detachment, vitritis, retinitis, choroiditis, vasculitis, perivasculitis and anterior chamber infiltration of varying intensity are commonly observed. Additional characteristics include iritis, scleritis, granuloma formation, and more rarely the appearance of Dalen-Fuchs nodules and subretinal neovascularization (Figure 5.1). For a detailed description of the pathology of EAU in its various forms, and a comparison with the human uveitic conditions that it is considered to represent, the interested reader is referred to the excellent reviews by Faure[1] and by Gery et al.[2].

EAU IN ANIMAL MODELS

Rodent models of EAU have been developed in the guinea pig, rat, rabbit and, more recently, the mouse. Differences have been noted in the uveitogenic responses of the various species. The reasons for these differences are not well understood; however, some of them might be due to fairly straightforward anatomical differences, such as the lack of retinal vessels in guinea pigs. Although none of the animal models of EAU reproduces the full spectrum of human uveitis, each model offers some unique properties, making it suitable for the study of specific aspects of ocular inflammatory disease.

Guinea pig

The guinea pig was the first animal in which ocular autoimmunity was successfully induced. These studies were pioneered by Collins[3], Aronson[4-6] and by Wacker and Lipton[7]. An exceptionally wide spectrum of clinical and histopathological features can be induced in this species, depending on the identity of the antigen, dose and route of immunization. By varying these parameters, disease course from chronic (over 1 year duration) to hyperacute can be observed[1,2]. In the less-than-hyperacute forms, pathology is concentrated mainly in the choroid, probably owing to the lack of retinal blood vessels in this species.

Rabbit

EAU in rabbits has been less thoroughly characterized than in other species; however, uveitogenic responses to retinal extracts as well as to purified retinal antigens have been reported[8-10].

Rat

Currently, the rat is used most widely as an EAU model. EAU in the Lewis rat is an acute disease that appears 12–16 days after immunization, and is characterized by an explosive, relatively short course, having an active phase of 1–2 weeks[1,2]. Typical acute-phase pathology takes on the appearance of panuveitis, with a heavy inflammatory cell infiltrate in the anterior chamber and the vitreous. Retinal pathology includes widespread detachment with infiltration of leukocytes into the subretinal space and massive photoreceptor destruction (Figure 5.1 (A)). A rat EAU model of a milder and more chronic nature has been described in the PVG rat[11] and more recently also in the Lister black hooded rat[12]. However, these alternative rat models have not yet gained wide acceptance.

Mouse

Until recently, mice have been considered a species refractory to EAU. However, use of an intensified immunization protocol and the use of the recently identified retinal uveitogen IRBP (interphotoreceptorretinoid-binding protein), has enabled the induction of EAU in several strains of mice[13]. The ability to mount a uveitogenic response was exhibited by a minority of the strains and appears to be at least in part dependent on the

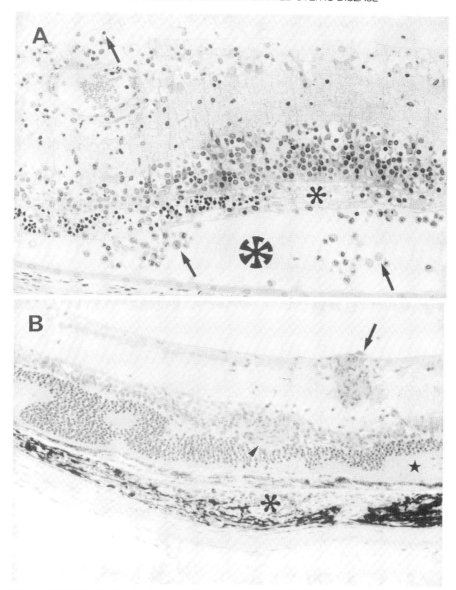

Figure 5.1 EAU pathology in the rat and mouse models. (A) SAg-EAU in the Lewis rat. Disease was induced by immunization with 30 μg of SAg in CFA. Eyes were processed for histopathology 2 weeks after immunization. Note serous retinal detachment (wheel), infiltrating inflammatory cells in the subretinal space and the retina (arrows) and extensive photoreceptor destruction (asterisk). (Haematoxylin and eosin, × 315). (B) IRBP-EAU in the B10.A mouse. Disease was induced with 100 μg of IRBP in CFA, given in two divided doses, with *B. pertussis* vaccine as additional adjuvant[12]. Eyes were processed 4 weeks after immunization. Note vasculitis (arrow), retinal granuloma (arrowhead), choroiditis (asterisk) and retinal fold with focal detachments (star). Photoreceptor cell layer is relatively well-preserved. (Haemotoxylin and eosin, × 225).

major histocompatibility complex (see "Genetic basis of susceptibility to EAU", below). In contrast, all strains studied were able to mount antibody and lymphocyte responses against the immunizing retinal antigen. Of the two retinal antigens studied, SAg (retinal soluble antigen) appears to be a less potent uveitogen in mice than IRBP[13]. IRBP uveitis in the B10.A mouse is a relatively chronic disease, starting during the third week after immunization and remaining active for a number of weeks. Damage to the retina and uvea is typically focal, with granuloma formation and vasculitis as prominent features (Figure 5.1B). Formation of Dalen–Fuchs nodules and subretinal neovascularization occur in a proportion of the animals. Vitritis and anterior chamber involvement are typically minimal[13]. Recent data suggest that in contrast to EAU in other rodents, murine EAU may be a relapsing disease (Chan and Caspi, submitted).

Primates

For obvious reasons, uveitis in primates is the closest model to ocular inflammation in the human. EAU in primates has been induced both with SAg and IRBP, raising the possibility that these retinal antigens may be involved also in human disease. Monkey EAU has a chronic course that lasts for many months and the lesions are reminiscent of several human ocular inflammatory diseases, primarily sympathetic ophthalmia, VKH and birdshot retinochoroidopathy[14–17]. Immunized monkeys exhibit both humoral and cellular responses to the immunizing antigen. In SAg-induced disease, Nussenblatt et al. reported mainly retinal involvement[15,16], while IRBP-induced disease appeared to affect mainly the choroid[14].

RETINAL ANTIGENS

Retinal extracts induce EAU when injected in emulsion with CFA into susceptible animals. At least three different uveitogenic proteins have been identified in these extracts and found to be able to induce EAU when used in their purified form, and there are indications that additional uveitogens are yet to be identified[2,10].

Retinal soluble antigen

Retinal soluble antigen (SAg) was the first uveitogen to be purified and characterized. This intracellular protein is a major component of rod outer segments, and is also found in the pineal gland[18,19]. Although there was some controversy as to the identity and biological function of this protein (see review by Gery et al.[2]), it has now been identified by Pfister et al. as the 48 kDa protein that participates in light-signal transduction[20]. SAg is a potent uveitogen in all the animal models thus far studied, with the possible exception of the mouse, of which a highly susceptible strain has yet to be identified[13]. A finding of potential significance is that some uveitis patients exhibit immunological responses to SAg[21]. It is not clear, however, whether this responsiveness is a primary phenomenon implicated in pathogenesis, or secondary autoimmunization to antigens released from damaged tissue.

Probably owing to its central role in the visual process, SAg appears to be an evolutionarily conserved molecule. A high degree of homology in the amino-acid sequence has been found in SAg from several mammalian species[22-24], and antigenic cross-reactivity has been reported with "SAg" of lower vertebrates and even invertebrates[25,26].

Cleavage fragments of bovine SAg have been used to identify regions in the molecule that contain structures involved in EAU induction[27,28]. By combining the information from fragment analysis and amino-acid sequence, Donoso and his associates[29,30] have synthesized a series of peptides around 20 amino acids each in length, three of which were identified as pathogenic in the rat EAU model (peptides K, N and M)[30,31]. Peptide M was found to be uveitogenic also in guinea pigs[32], which contrasts with findings in a variety of other autoantigens, where recognition of pathogenic sites was found to be uniquely species- and even strain-specific. Epitopes derived from the human SAg sequence that were identified as pathogenic in the rat correspond to the bovine M and N peptides[33]. All the uveitogenic epitopes reside in a relatively small segment of the C-terminal half of the SAg molecule. None of the three peptides possesses the full pathogenicity of SAg, which might indicate the lack of immunodominance on behalf of the pathogenic epitopes they contain. On a molar basis, immunization with much higher amounts of the peptides than the intact SAg molecule is needed to induce EAU, and a uveitogenic rat T-helper lymphocyte line specific to SAg does not show detectable proliferation with any of these peptides (Caspi, unpublished). In contrast, larger cyanogen bromide fragments of SAg are recognized by T-helper lines specific to SAg[34]. These results suggest that there is at least one other pathogenic determinant in the SAg molecule yet to be characterized, which might perhaps constitute the immunodominant epitope.

Interphotoreceptor retinoid binding protein (IRBP)

IRBP is a 140 kDa glycoprotein whose physiological role in the retina is believed to be in the transport of vitamin A derivatives between the retinal pigment epithelium and the photoreceptors[35]. In keeping with its biological function, IRBP is primarily an extracellular protein[36]. Similarly to SAg, IRBP appears to be an evolutionarily conserved molecule[37,38]. In addition to being found in the retina, IRBP is also found in the pineal gland, and small amounts were detected in the brain cortex[39,40]. Minor differences were reported in the course, immunopathology and immunogenetics of EAU induced in rats by bovine IRBP in comparison to EAU induced by SAg[41-43]. Similarly to SAg, IRBP induces EAU also in rabbits[9] and primates[14]. In contrast to SAg, IRBP is poorly pathogenic in guinea pigs[44], but in mice it was found to be more a potent immunopathogen than SAg[13].

The approach to delineating the pathogenic epitopes of bovine IRBP has been similar to the strategy employed in defining the pathogenic epitopes of SAg. After defining the pathogenic regions of IRBP from cyanogen bromide cleavage fragments, and utilizing the known amino-acid sequence, short stretches of the molecule were synthesized and tested for pathogenicity in rats[45,46]. Thus far, two pathogenic epitopes that induce EAU in the rat were identified in the bovine IRBP molecule. One of these epitopes is included in peptides R4 and R9 (ref. 46 and I. Gery, in press), which share a stretch of homology. This epitope appears not to be immunodominant, in the sense that higher quauntities of peptide than of whole IRBP on a molar basis are required to induce disease, and lymph node cells of rats immunized with the whole molecule do not proliferate to the peptide, and vice versa. Another peptide, designated R14, contains a uveitogenic epitope localized to a minimal sequence of 11 amino acids, and appears to be an immunodominant epitope of IRBP, inducing EAU in submicrogram quantities and showing immunological crossreactivity with the whole IRBP molecule (ref. 47 and I. Gery, in press). Not surprisingly, both epitopes that were pathogenic rats were not pathogenic in mice (Caspi, unpublished). Several epitopes in the human IRBP molecule that induced EAU in the rat were recently identified by Donoso et al.[48].

Rhodopsin

The uveitogenic potential of rhodopsin, and its illuminated form opsin, has been somewhat controversial because of a possible contamination of the preparations with SAg[2]. However, EAU has been obtained with highly purified preparations of this protein in the guinea pig as well as in the rat[49-52]. The pathogenicity of this molecule appears to be conformation-dependent, since opsin was shown to be considerably less pathogenic than rhodopsin[53].

IMMUNOPATHOLOGICAL AND REGULATORY MECHANISMS IN EAU

Cellular mechanisms in EAU induction and pathogenesis

Current knowledge indicates that cell-mediated immunity plays a major role in the induction of experimental ocular autoimmune disease. It has been known for a long time that development of EAU is invariably linked to development of delayed-type hypersensitivity (DTH) to the immunizing retinal antigen. Moreover, EAU can be transferred to naive animals with lymphocytes, but not serum, of genetically identical donors immunized with a retinal antigen[54-56]. The capacity to transfer disease resides in a lymphocyte fraction enriched for the T-helper/inducer subset, and T-suppressor/cytotoxic lymphocytes are incapable of disease transfer[56]. Direct evidence implicating T-helper lymphocytes in EAU induction was provided by the finding that EAU could be adoptively transferred with long-term T cell lines derived from rats immunized with SAg[34,57,58]. All the T-cell lines capable of adoptively transferring EAU that have been developed by different investigators, are antigen-specific and MHC Class II-restricted. All are of the helper/inducer phenotype (CD4+) and mediate DTH at the same time as they mediate EAU.

The use of in vivo functional, long-term T lymphocyte lines for the study of cellular mechanisms involved in EAU presents obvious advantages, since these lines represent readily available, homogeneous populations of cells, which easily lend themselves to characterization and manipulation. One such lymphocyte line, the ThS line, developed in our laboratory by a process of simultaneous selection for antigen specificity and for helper phenotypes from Lewis rats primed with SAg[58], has been used extensively in such studies, and has provided answers to a variety of basic questions.

The uveitgenic T-helper lymphocytes, as represented by the ThS and similar long-term lines, are probably not the actual cells that mediate histopathological damage. Rather, they appear to recruit host-derived mononuclear and polymorphonuclear effector cells, and to convey specificity to the pathogenic process. There are several lines of evidence that lend support to this interpretation. Radioactively labelled ThS cells injected systemically into a nonimmune animal do not measurably accumulate in the eye, while nevertheless inducing EAU[59]. This in itself suggests the participation of some amplification mechanism. In locally induced EAU, when line cells are placed directly in the vitreous cavity of the eye, relatively small numbers migrate into the retina and the onset of photoreceptor damage coincides with the influx of host-derived leukocytes entering the eye from the circulation[60,61]. Intravitreal transfer of activated lymphocytes that do not recognize a retinal antigen is also followed by influx of host cells. However, in the latter case, there is no preferential damage to photoreceptors, suggesting the need for *in situ* antigen recognition as an element of specificity[58,61]. Recruitment of the other T cells by the uveitogenic lymphocytes may be an important factor in the amplification of the inflammatory process. Systemic adoptive transfer of the uveitogenic ThS line into nude rats, which congenitally lack a thymus and have no endogenous T cells, does not result in EAU induction unless the nude animal is reconstituted with lymphocytes from a euthymic donor (Caspi, unpublished). Since partially selected T cell populations from SAg-primed donors are able to adoptively transfer EAU to nude rats[62], it is conceivable that at least one of the cells necessary for EAU development is a non-antigen-specific T cell. Taken together, these results indicate a central role for cell recruitment in the pathogenesis of EAU.

It is significant that, in order to effectively mediate EAU, the uveitogenic T cells must be stimulated with the specific antigen or with a T-cell mitogen, just prior to transfer. The reason for this requirement is not well understood, but it may in part be related to activation of mechanisms necessary for recruitment of host-derived effector cells, such as the secretion of various lymphokines. Activated, but not rested, ThS cells secrete interleukin-2 (IL-2), interleukin-3 (IL-3), interferon-gamma (IFN-γ), and macrophage-chemotactic activity (ref. 63 and Caspi, unpublished). Another function that is activated in helper T-cells by antigenic stimulation is the secretion of matrix-degrading enzymes such as heparan sulphate endoglycosidase, which may facilitate extravasation and penetration into the target organ[64].

How the autoimmune lymphocytes are able to "identify" their target organ from within the circulation is still an open question in organ-specific autoimmune lymphocytes to leave the circulation and accumulate in the eye[59,65]. Chronic *in situ* presentation of autoanitgens by organ resident cells, released from damaged photoreceptor tissue, seems to constitute a signal for autoimmune lymphocytes to leave the circulation and accumulate in eye[59,65]. Chronic *in situ* presentation of autoantigens by organ resident cells, aberrantly expressing MHC Class II, has been implicated in fuelling autoimmune inflammation in several organ-specific autoimmune diseases[66-68]. However, under conditions of EAU induction by adoptive transfer of ThS cells into a naive host, the uveitogenic lymphocyte encounters an intact eye without detectable tissue MHC Class II expression or antigen release. It is the personal bias of this author that, in the healthy host, extravasation of lymphocytes from the bloodstream into the tissues occurs at random. However, the occasional SAg-specific lymphocytes that pass through the retinal vasculature and "wander" into the eye would be able to initiate a chain of pathological events there that could not take place in another organ, because of the presence of the specific antigen at that location. A putative scenario would include induction of MHC Class II antigens by the locally secreted IFN-γ on nearby organ-resident cells, such as adjacent RPE and neighbouring vascular endothelial cells, and infiltration into the eye of the first leukocytes attracted by secreted lymphokines. RPE cells, which normally phagocytize and digest rod outer segments, might be able to act as antigen-presenting cells once MHC Class II antigens have been induced. In addition, initial focal damage to photoreceptor cells may already be occurring at this point by activated oxygen products produced by the infiltrating leukocytes[69,70], releasing free antigen. Local presentation of antigen released from the damaged photoreceptors, providing a continuing source of stimulation to uveitogenic T-helper cells, would serve to rapidly amplify the pathological process. This proposed sequence of events is in keeping with the previously mentioned data of Lightman et al.[59], who showed that EAU is initiated in the absence of measurable homing of ThS lymphocytes to the eye, and with experimental evidence showing that MHC Class II on ocular tissues is induced early in the EAU process, preceding or coinciding with the appearance of detectable inflammation[60,71,72].

The role of antibodies

The role of antibodies in EAU remains undefined. Although high titres of antibodies to SAg are induced concurrently with EAU in immunized animals, full-blown EAU can be induced (by adoptive transfer) without the presence of any detectable serum antibody[56,58]. Conversely, EAU can be suppressed (by cyclosporin A treatment) without apparent decrease in the titre of serum antibodies to SAg[73], and systemic injection of hyperimmune serum from SAg-immunized animals does not result in EAU induction[54,55]. Furthermore, although depletion of serum complement by cobra venom factor has been reported to reduce EAU intensity in SAg-immunized guinea pigs[74], McMaster et al. showed that NIH strain guinea pigs lacking the fourth component of complement were as susceptible to EAU as those with the enzyme[75]. It would therefore appear that humoral immunity is not mandatory to the disease. However, some experimental results suggest that serum antibodies may play an auxiliary role in modulating EAU either in the positive or in the negative direction, depending on their subclass and specificity.

In guinea pigs, injection of hyperimmune sera to rod outer segments directly into the eye can elicit EAU-like pathology[76]. Antibodies of the IgE subclass (reaginic) are detectable in rats immunized with SAg before the onset of EAU, and might mediate the mast cell degranulation that occurs shortly

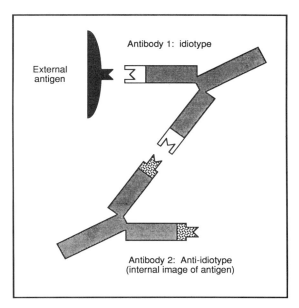

Figure 5.2 Idiotypic specificity. The active site of the antiidiotypic antibody is similar in structure to the original eliciting antigen.

before disease onset[77]. Release of vasoactive amines contained in the mast cell granules may contribute to EAU induction by increasing the permeability of ocular blood vessels. In support of this theory is the observation that sensitivity to EAU of different rat strains appears to be correlated with the number of choroidal mast cells[78], and that local treatment with pharmacological agents that block mast cell function can delay or suppress EAU[79].

Recent experimental evidence suggests that antibodies of antiidiotypic specificity may be implicated in the negative regulation of EAU[80]. Immunization of rats with monoclonal mouse antibodies to SAg results in the formation of anti-antibodies, some of which will recognize the hypervariable domain (idiotype) of the immunizing antibody molecule. Since antigen and the active site of the specific antibody complement each other in structure, the antiidiotypic antibodies that are directed to the antigen-binding site would mimic an epitope on SAg that is recognized by the original monoclonal antibody (Figure 5.2). De Kozak and her collaborators have demonstrated that immunization of rats with monoclonals to certain epitopes of SAg results in protection from EAU inducted by a subsequent challenge with the whole SAg molecule.

Idiotypic networks, in which each idiotype in its turn elicits an antiidiotypic response, have been proposed to constitute a major mechanism that might control immune responses[81]. The mechanism of resistance to EAU by idiotype immunization is unknown. Current knowledge indicates that antibody-recognized epitopes are usually different from T-cell-recognized epitopes, and it is the latter that should be implicated in EAU. However, direct induction of cellular immunity by antiidotype immunization has been reported in the case of a reovirus antigen, where T and B cells appear to share idiotypic configurations[82]. Antiidiotypic antibodies that present an "internal image" of a pathogenic site of SAg could thus be theorized to "block" the antigen receptors of uveitogenic T cells. Alternatively, it is conceivable that idiotype immunization might be initiating a regulatory circuit, resulting in the induction of antiidiotypic T-suppressor cells, in parallel to antiidiotypic antibodies. In the model of experimental autoimmune encephalomyelitis (EAE), in which immunopathogenic mechanisms are similar to those in EAU, antiidiotypic suppressor cells that recognize the antigen receptor of an encephalitogenic T cell clone are able to protect rats from disease induced by adoptive transfer of the same clone[83]. Participation of suppressor cells in the downregulation of EAU in the rat has been suggested on the basis of results showing *in vivo* suppression of the disease by a long-term T-cell line with suppressor function derived from SAg primed donors[84] (see below).

Suppressor T cells in EAU

The evidence linking suppressor T cells to the negative regulation of experimental ocular autoimmunity is derived mostly from studies in the rat model. Chan et al.[85,86] have shown a direct correlation between the increase in the eye of the number of lymphocytes bearing the suppressor/cytotoxic membrane marker OX8 (the rat equivalent of CD8), and termination of the active stage of EAU. Moreover, in EAU induced by IRBP, OX8+ cells appear in the eye sooner than in EAU induced by SAg, and this coincides with a shorter course of the IRBP-induced disease[87]. Conversely, relative lack of cells bearing suppressor/cytotoxic markers in murine EAU correlates with a prolonged and possibly relapsing form of disease (Chan and Caspi, submitted). In the absence of any evidence pointing to a role for cytotoxic T cells in EAU, these results must be interpreted as strongly suggestive of suppressor cell involvement in the downregulation of the disease process. Fujino *et al.* showed that rats primed with SAg and protected from EAU development by a short course of treatment with cyclosporin A develop a specific unresponsiveness to a second challenge with SAg[88]. Lymphocyte fractions enriched in suppressor cells that were isolated from these rats suppressed proliferation of SAg-primed lymphocytes to SAg *in vitro*, and inhibited or delayed the development of EAU when adoptively transferred to recipient rats immunized with S-antigen.

The most direct evidence to date, linking suppressor T cells to the negative regulation of EAU, is the observation that a long-term lymphocyte live with suppressor function can downregulate EAU *in vivo*[84]. This cell line was derived from rats primed with SAg in the anterior chamber of the eye (a regimen that under certain conditions can result in preferential induction of suppression rather than help[89]) after *in vitro* restimulation with the specific antigen and selection for the suppressor (OX8+) phenotype. The inhibitory function of the resultant cell line was both antigen-non-specific and radio-resistant, properties consistent with a terminally differentiated population of suppressor cells[90]. Since this *in vivo* functional suppressor line could inhibit primed T-helper cells, such as would be present during the expression stage of disease, it was suggested that efferent-acting T-suppressor cells may play a role in the downregulation of EAU[84].

In addition to suppressor T cells, other regulatory mechanisms may participate in the suppression or prevention of EAU. A possible role for antiidiotypic antibodies in the suppression of EAU has already been mentioned (see preceding section).

Ocular resident cells as locally acting suppressor cells

A possible role for non-lymphoid ocular-resident cells in the negative regulation of EAU has been proposed on the basis of interactions between retinal glial cells (Müller cells) and lymphocytes, as studied in an *in vitro* system derived from the rat model of EAU. Müller cells isolated from the retina proliferate in culture in the presence of lymphokines released from activated lymphocytes/monocytes, and supernatants from the uveitogenic ThS lymphocytes are particularly efficient at stimulating Müller cell growth[91]. However, when Müller cells are co-cultured with ThS cells, they profoundly suppress proliferation, IL-2 production and IL-2 receptor expression of ThS responding to antigen (presented on conventional antigen-presenting cells), and also suppress their subsequent IL-2-dependent proliferation[92]. The suppression was shown to affect T-helper cells of different antigenic specificities, and to require direct contact between Müller cells and ThS cells. On the basis of these findings, and in view of numerous reported observations that Müller cells are spared or even proliferate in a variety of ocular inflammatory conditions, it seems plausible that a putative equivalent of these interactions *in vivo* might serve as a local mechanism that could downregulate ocular inflammation.

Interestingly, Müller cells that are made to express MHC Class II in the course of culture with IFN-γ-containing supernatants, are fully capable of acting as antigen-presenting cells to the uveitogenic ThS, cells if the membrane-bound inhibitor is removed by a treatment with trypsin, and prevented from being resynthesized by chemical fixation of the cell membrane with glutaraldehyde[93]. The significance of this finding with respect to a potential *in vivo* role of Müller cells as local antigen-presenting cells is unknown, since under "physiological" culture conditions the suppressive function of the Müller cells completely overrides their potential to present antigen. Local presentation of antigen by organ-resident cells aberrantly expressing MHC Class II has been implicated in autoimmune phenomena[66-68]. It is conceivable that suppressive mechanisms such as this might have evolved in order to prevent some organ-resident cells with the potential to present antigen, such as the Müller cell, from initiating and perpetuating autoimmunity.

GENETIC BASIS OF SUSCEPTIBILITY TO EAU

A strong association between genetic background and the propensity to develop particular kinds of autoimmune disease has been demonstrated in a variety of experimental and clinical situations (for reviews see refs. 94, 95, 96). In human uveitis, Nussenblatt *et al.* have shown a strong association between HLA-A29 and birdshot retinochoroidopathy, and found responsiveness to SAg in these patients[97]. Genetic control of EAU has been documented; however, its immunogenetics have not been studied in depth owing to the lack, until recently, of an EAU model in a genetically well-characterized species.

McMaster *et al.* studied EAU induction with retinal and uveal antigens in several strains of guinea pigs[75]. The Hartley and NIH strains could be classified as high responders, strain 13 animals could be classified as intermediate responders, and strain 2 guinea pigs were non-responders. Control of EAU in rats by genes of the major histocompatibility complex has been suggested by the studies of Gery and his collaborators. Rats of the RT1^l haplotype, Lewis and CAR, were high responders to SAg-induced EAU, while rats of several other haplotypes were low responders or non-responders[2]. Fisher 344 rats, which have a slightly modified RT1^l haplotype, had uveitogenic and immunological response patterns identical to those of Lewis rats to the epitope contained in peptide R14 of IRBP, while different recognition patterns and lack of uveitogenic response were exhibited by strains of other RT1 haplotypes[47]. In mice, out of a variety of haplotypes tested, the uveitogenic response has so far been found only in strains of the H-2^k haplotype, and in related strains carrying the H-2^k serological specificity in the IA (and the K) region of the H-2[13]. Curiously, none of these strains have developed EAU in response to both SAg and IRBP. Rather, the uveitogenic response to these two antigens appeared to be mutually exclusive. Susceptibility to either SAg or IRBP of mouse strains sharing the same H-2 haplotype suggests not only intra- but also extra-MHC control of susceptibility to EAU in mice.

Extra-MHC control of EAU induction might include genetic factors connected to local vasoactive amine release, and therefore to changes in the permeability of blood vessels in the target organ. Susceptibility to EAE in mice is controlled by a combined effect of H-2 and histamine-sensitization genes[98]. In the rat EAU model, Mochizuki *et al.*[78] found a correlation in several strains between their number of choroidal mast cells and their susceptibility to disease. A case in point is the low susceptibility to EAU exhibited by the LeR strain. LeR is an EAE-resistant mutant of Lewis, whose loss of susceptibility to autoimmune disease is still unexplained[99,100]. The number of choroidal mast cells in LeR was found to be only one-quarter of those in Lewis rats. In view of the evidence that vasoactive amines released by choroidal mast cells may facilitate EAU development[77,79], these investigators proposed that the reduced number of mast cells in LeR and some other rat strains could be responsible for their lowered susceptibility to EAU. Evidence in support of this interpretation is provided by the finding that treatment of LeR rats with *Bordetella pertussis* adjuvant converts them to high responders[78]. Pertussis adjuvant may act by increasing the sensitivity of vascular endothelial cells to vasoactive amines, as suggested on the basis of results obtained in the mouse EAE model[101].

Another genetic characteristic that might affect susceptibility to autoimmune disease could be differences in the ability to upregulate tissue MHC Class II expression in response to an immunological challenge. Wilder *et al.* noted a pronounced difference in this respect in rats of the Lewis and F344 strains (which share a closely related MHC haplotype) that was correlated with the susceptibility of these two strains to develop streptococcal cell wall-induced arthritis. While tissue-specific MHC Class II expression in the Lewis was strongly upregulated and severe arthritis was induced, F344 animals showed minimal induction of MHC Class II in the tissue and minimal or no arthritis[102]. We noted a similar difference between these two strains in their susceptibility to SAg-induced EAU[103]. Interestingly, LeR rats in the same study were susceptible to SAg-EAU without the use of pertussis adjuvant. This is at variance with results previously reported by Mochizuki *et al.*[78], and could be due to a genetic drift occurring over time in individual rat colonies. Quantitative evaluation of choroidal mast cells in the susceptible LeR should be done, and might yield interesting results.

IMMUNOTHERAPY OF EAU

In addition to providing a model for the study of basic immunological mechanisms in ocular inflammation, EAU also provides a means of testing the efficacy of various treatment modalities. In recent years, attention has centred on various immunomodulatory agents as a means to control immune-mediated inflammatory processes in the eye. The aim is to achieve specificity in immunosuppression, so as to affect the processes involved in immunopatho-genesis, while causing minimal suppression of the immune response in general. The treatments that could be predicted to be most effective in counteracting immunopathogenic mechanisms such as the ones represented by EAU would be the ones affecting the cellular, rather than the humoral, arm of the immune response. In addition, any treatment of practical value would have to be effective during the efferent stage of disease, paralleling the clinical situation in which pre-existing inflammation is present.

Immunosuppressive drugs

A major breakthrough in the treatment of uveitic diseases, that stemmed directly from experiments performed in the EAU model, has been the introduction of cyclosporin A (CsA) as a therapeutic modality[73,104,105]. CsA treatment can prevent EAU when started either during the afferent (days 0–7) or during the efferent (days 7–14) stages of EAU; however, increased doses are needed if the beginning of treatment is delayed[73,106]. CsA (a fungal-derived cyclic endecapeptide) is considered to be primarily a T-cell inhibitor that preferentially suppresses activation and proliferation of T-helper and T-cytotoxic lymphocytes with a relative sparing of T-suppressor cells (for reviews see Shevach[107] and Hess *et al.*[108]). In SAg-immunized rats treated with cyclosporin, the cellular responses to SAg and the number of T-helper/inducer cells in the draining lymph nodes are greatly reduced[109,110]. It is therefore a reasonable conclusion that inhibition of the clonal expansion of uveitogenic T-helper lymphocytes, combined with the sparing of specific T-suppressor lymphocytes[88], may be the underlying mechanism in EAU suppression. The effects of CsA on several activation parameters of the uveitogenic ThS lymphocyte line suggest that this inhibition is a composite of several effects, including suppression of IL-2 production, inhibition of IL-2 receptor expression and a block of proliferation by an additional, as yet uncharacterized, mechanism[111].

CsA is a cytostatic agent whose effects on lymphocytes are reversible. Moreover, triggering of the pathogenic potential of uveitogenic T lymphocytes can apparently occur despite the presence of CsA, to become manifest as soon as the drug is withdrawn[111]. It is therefore not surprising that lasting suppression of disease requires continuous cyclosporin treatment[106,112,113].

A major problem in the prolonged clinical use of CsA has been its pronounced nephrotoxic effect[113]. Topical treatment with CsA was found to be ineffective, owing to the lack of penetration of the drug into the globe[114]. This brought about the search for a suitable substitute, or an additive that would permit reduction of the dosage. A number of other agents, such as steroids, cytotoxic drugs and other immunosuppressive agents, were tested and found to be inferior to cyclosporin in the EAU model[115–118]. Furthermore, none of these substitutes could suppress EAU without also affecting humoural immunity. In contrast, efficient suppression of EAU by FK-506, a new immunosuppressive drug with an *in vivo* mode of action apparently similar to that of cyclosporin, has recently been reported by Kawashima *et al.*[119]. A potentially promising treatment alternative that has recently been under investigation is the use of natural or synthetic CsA analogues. Both cyclosporin G and cyclosporin D have been found effective in suppressing EAU, and in inhibiting proliferation of uveitogenic T-helper cells in the rat model[120]. However, in comparison to CsA, larger doses of CsG, and considerably larger doses of CsD, were required to achieve a similar effect, a problem that may well outweigh any relative reduction in toxicity. A definitive answer to this question awaits further clinical trials.

A novel approach to the enhancement of cyclosporin therapy has been initiated by Palestine *et al.*[121]. Since cyclosporin and prolactin appear to compete for the same binding site on lymphoid cells[122], these investigators used bromocriptine (a dopamine receptor agonist that inhibits pituitary prolactin secretion) in a combination treatment with cyclosporin, in order to achieve the same therapeutic effects with lower cyclosporin doses. The bromocriptine–cyclosporin combination treatment, shown to be effective in the rat EAU model[121], has subsequently yielded encouraging preliminary results in a clinical trial with a small number of uveitis patients[123]. It remains to be seen whether this approach will indeed result in long-term treatment benefits.

Monoclonal antibodies and receptor-targeting strategies

Another solution to achieving selective immunosuppression in EAU therapy is being explored through the use of monoclonal antibodies. Knowledge of the basic mechanisms of the induction and pathogenesis of EAU suggests that various monoclonal reagents could be useful in an attempt to interrupt the disease process at different stages. For example, monoclonal antibodies to MHC Class II antigens could interfere with the process of antigen presentation, and suppress the activity of MHC Class II-positive lymphocytes and monocytes. Treatment with anti-T-cell antibodies could preferentially suppress the cellular arm of the immune response, leaving humoral immunity relatively unaffected. Treatment with anti-MHC Class II antibodies was shown to suppress development of EAE in the mouse model[124]. Wetzig *et al.* have presented evidence that such treatment may also downgrade EAU induction in the rat[125]. Recent data indicate that treatment with antibody to the T-helper marker W3/25 may also be beneficial in this model (Higuchi and Caspi, in preparation).

Immunotherapy of EAU by immunization of rats with mouse monoclonals specific to certain (immunopathogenic?) epitopes of the SAg molecule was employed by de Kozak *et al.*[80]. The significance of this treatment in eliciting protective antiidiotypic antibodies, and possibly antiidiotypic suppressor mechanisms, has already been discussed in the section that deals with the role of antibodies in EAU.

Higuchi *et al.* used monoclonal anti-IL-2 receptor antibodies in an attempt to target activated (IL-2 receptor expressing) uveitogenic lymphocytes. Optimal results in the treatment of the efferent stage of rat EAU, represented by adoptive transfer of ThS lymphocytes, were obtained by a combination therapy with ART18 (a mouse monoclonal recognizing the IL-2-binding site of the rat IL-2 receptor[126]) and low-dose cyclosporin[127]. Most of the animals treated with the combination therapy were protected from EAU, and animals treated with ART18 alone were partially protected. Splenocytes of protected animals did not transfer EAU to untreated recipients, suggesting elimination or inactivation of the uveitogenic lymphocytes by the treatment.

Another way of targeting IL-2-receptor-bearing lymphocytes has been employed by Roberge *et al.*[128]. These investigators used a genetically engineered chimeric toxin, composed of IL-2 fused to a modified pseudomonas exotoxin lacking its cell-recognition domain[129]. The bound IL-2 toxin is internalized by receptor-mediated endocytosis, whereupon the toxin kills the cell. Lewis rats actively immunized with SAg and treated with the toxin during the efferent stage of disease showed reduced incidence and severity of EAU, as well as a net reduction in the T-cell population of IL-2 receptor-bearing cells. However, before any therapy relying on treatment with xenogeneic monoclonal antibodies, or with engineered toxins containing bacterial proteins, can be successfully transplanted to the clinic, the problem of the immunological response of the host to the treatment will have to be addressed[127].

An approach of considerable ingenuity and therapeutic potential is immunization against idiotypic determinants of the antigen receptor of (autologous) autoimmune T-helper cells. This method of 'T-cell vaccination', which apparently results in the activation of antiiodiotypic suppressor cells, has been successful in suppressing several organ-specific autoimmune diseases in rats and in mice[83,130,131]. Although a parallel approach to immunotherapy of EAU has so far yielded equivocal results (Gery, personal communication and Caspi, unpublished), this line of investigation merits further experimentation.

Enhancement of suppressor mechanisms by feeding with antigen

Presentation of antigens through the gut has been shown in a variety of systems to result in the induction of active antigen-specific suppression that effectively inhibits both primary and established immune responses[132–135]. Feeding of rats with myelin basic protein suppresses development of EAE when administered either before or after immunization[136,137]. Nusenblatt et al. have fed Lewis rats with soluble SAg or bovine serum albumin (BSA). The SAg-fed animals, but not the BSA-fed animals, were protected from development of EAU after a subsequent challenge with SAg. Spleen cells from these animals suppressed in vitro antigen- and mitogen-driven proliferation of the SAg-specific uveitogenic ThS line. Splenocytes of SAg-fed animals contained antigen-specific suppressive activity, attributable to OX8+ cells, as well as antigen-non-specific activity, while splenocytes of BSA-fed donors could effect only antigen-non-specific suppression (Nussenblatt, Caspi et al., submitted).

Enchancement of natural suppressive mechanisms by a treatment that is easily applied and presents no hazard to the patient is an extremely attractive therapeutic approach. However, although some uveitis patients exhibit immunological responses to SAg[21,97], the eliciting antigens in human uveitis have not yet been identified. Additional studies that might help to elucidate this important question are urgently needed.

OTHER (NON-EAU) MODELS OF OCULAR INFLAMMATION

This review would not be complete without a brief mention of other, non-EAU, models of immune-mediated ocular inflammation.

Endotoxin (LPS)-induced uveitis

Endotoxin-induced uveitis in rabbits and in rats is primarily a model of anterior uveitis, and has been suggested to have relevance to human disease[138]. LPS uveitis is elicited by a single intravitreal or systemic injection of endotoxin[139,140]. The inflammatory response is rapid (induced within several hours) and brief (lasting several days)[140]. The inflammatory process involves a breakdown of the blood–aqueous barrier, with influx of protein and cells into the anterior chamber[140]. The mediators that have been directly implicated in these phenomena include arachidonic acid metabolites (primarily PGE2), as well as macrophage- and neutrophil-chemotactic activities, all of which can be demonstrated in the anterior chamber fluid[141–145]. Tissue MHC Class II expression is induced early in the inflammation, but its significance is unknown[146]. The active moiety in the endotoxin molecule appears to be lipid A[144,147].

It is believed that the mode of action of LPS in the eye may involve its well-documented ability to stimulate production of cytokines such as interleukin-1 (IL-1) and tumour necrosis factor (TNF). However, the notion that TNF is the primary inducer in LPS uveitis has recently been challenged by Rosenbaum *et al.*, who found differences between uveitis caused by injection of recombinant TNF and that caused by recombinant IL-1 or by endotoxin[148]. The mechanism of induction of ocular symptoms by systemically administered endotoxin is not well understood. Rosenbaum *et al.*[149] reported that systemically injected labelled LPS does not localize in ocular tissues, and suggested that the ocular effects are indirect. However, Howes *et al.*[150] were able to detect trace amounts of LPS in the ciliary processes and aqueous humour a short time after its systemic administration. In contrast, in anterior uveitis induced by systemic injection of streptococcal cell walls, bacterial components have been demonstrated in the eye, suggesting a "depot" mechanism of inflammation[151].

Immunogenic uveitis (albumin-induced uveitis)

This model of uveitis is considered primarily as a model of antibody-mediated disease; however, T cells may also participate in the pathogenesis of this model[152-154]. Inflammation is induced by hyperimmunizing animals with xenogeneic serum albumin, followed by an intravitreal challenge with the immunizing antigen at the peak of antibody production[153]. Severe uveitis is induced within 24 hours. Another regimen that has been used to induce immunogenic uveitis is injection of albumin into the vitreous of unprimed animals, resulting in a delayed induction of uveitis[155], coincident with the appearance of humoral antibodies. Intravenous challenge with the immunizing antigen at a later time causes a rapid re-induction of inflammation[155], suggesting prolonged persistence of the foreign albumin in the eye. Immune complexes are present in the aqueous humour during clinically evident inflammation, indicating involvement of complement activation[152]. Leukocyte-chemotactic activity, apparently similar to that in LPS-iduced uveitis, is present in the aqueous humour[155,156]. A role for arachidonic acid metabolites and for T-cell-derived lymphokines has also been suggested[154,157]. Curiously, even though this uveitis occurs in response to a non-ocular antigen, photoreceptor damage similar to that seen in EAU has been reported[153].

Lens-induced uveitis (LIU)

LIU in rodents serves as a model for human lens-induced uveitis (phakogenic uveitis) and is considered to be an immune-complex-mediated, Arthus-type reaction[158-160]. Immunity is induced by priming with xenogeneic lens proteins, and uveitis is subsequently precipitated by mechanical trauma to the lens. Immunization with lens proteins without mechanical disruption of the lens capsule does not result in uveitis, presumably because an intact lens capsule prevents antibody access to the source of autologous antigen. Typical LIU takes the form of granulomatous endophthalmitis[159,160]. As in other forms of acute uveitis accompanied by massive accumulation of inflammatory leukocytes, activated oxygen products and hydroxyl radicals appear to play an important role in tissue damage[161,162]. Arachidonic acid metabolites produced by the lipoxygenase pathway may also participate in the pathogenesis of LIU[163].

Cytokine-mediated ocular inflammation

A unique type of ocular inflammation, without a known parallel in naturally occurring disease, has been observed in transgenic mice that express the gene for granulocyte-macrophage colony-stimulating factor (GM-CSF), a haemopoietic growth factor. Early in life, the eyes of these mice develop accumulations of macrophages, cataracts and retinal damage[164]. These ocular findings are part of a more generalized, ultimately fatal, syndrome of tissue damage. The accumulation of activated macrophages in the eyes is apparently due to the transcription of the GM-CSF gene within the ocular tissue. It is conceivable that products such as oxygen radicals and TNF, released by the activated macrophages, could be directly responsible for the observed ocular pathology.

References

1. Faure, J. P. (1980). Autoimmunity and the retina. *Curr. Top. Eye Res.*, **2**, 215–301
2. Gery, I., Mochizuki, M. and Nussenblatt, R. B. (1986). Retinal specific antigens and immunopathogenic processes they provoke. *Prog. Retinal Res.*, **5**, 75–109
3. Collins, R. C. (1949). Experimental studies on sympathetic ophthalmia. *Am. J. Ophthalmol.*, **32**, 129–35
4. Aronson, S. B., Hogan, M. J. and Zweigart, P. (1983). Homoimmune uveitis in the guinea-pig. I. General concepts of auto- and homoimmunity, methods and manifestations. *Arch. Ophthalmol.*, **69**, 105–9
5. Aronson, S. B., Hogan, M. J. and Zweigart, P. (1963). Homoimmune uveitis in the guinea-pig. II. Clinical manifestations. *Arch. Ophthalmol.*, **69**, 203–7
6. Aronson, S. B., Hogan M. J. and Zweigart, P. (1963). Homoimmune uveitis in the guinea-pig. III. Histopathologic manifestations of the disease. *Arch. Ophthalmol.*, **69**, 208–19
7. Wacker, W. B. and Lipton, M. M. (1968). Experimental allergic uveitis. I. Production in the guinea-pig and rabbit by immunization with retina in adjuvant. *J. Immunol.*, **101**, 151–5
8. Rao, N. A., Brown, C. J. and Marak, G. E (1986). Untrastructural analysis of experimental allergic uveitis in rabbit. *Ophthalmic Res.*, **18**, 15–20
9. Eisenfield, A. J., Bunt-Milam, A. H. and Saari, J. C. (1987). Uveoretinitis in rabbits following immunization with interphotoreceptor retinoid-binding protein. *Exp. Eye Res.*, **44**, 425–38
10. Kalsow, C. M. and Wacker, W. B. (1986). Rabbit ocular and pineal autoimmune response to retina antigens. *Curr. Eye Res.*, **5**, 579–856
11. de Kozak, Y., Sakai, J., Thillaye, B. and Faure, J. P. (1981). S antigen-induced experimental autoimmune uveo-retinitis in rats. *Curr. Eye Res.*, **1**, 327–40
12. Stanford, M. R., Brown, E. C., Kasp, E., Graham, E. M., Sanders, M. D. and Dumonde, D. C. (1987). Experimental posterior uveitis. I: A clinical, angiographic, and pathological study. *Br. J. Ophthalmol.*, **71**, 585–92
13. Caspi, R. R., Roberge, F. G., Chan, C. C., Wiggert, B., Chader, G. J., Rozenszajn, L. A., Lando, Z. and Nussenblatt, R. B. (1988). A new model of autoimmune disease. Experimental autoimmune uveoretinitis induced in mice with two different retinal antigens. *J. Immunol.*, **140**, 1490–5
14. Hirose, S., Kuwabara, T., Nussenblatt, R. B., Wiggert, B., Redmond, T. M. and Gery, I. (1986). Uveitis induced in primates by interphotoreceptor retinoid-binding protein. *Arch. Ophthalmol.*, **104**, 1698–702
15. Nussenblatt, R. B., Kuwabara, T., de Monasterio, F. M. and Wacker, W. B. (1981). S-antigen uveitis in primates. A new model for human disease. *Arch. Ophthalmol.*, **99**, 1090–2

16. Hirose, S., Wiggert, B., Redmond, T. M., Kuwabara, T., Nussenblatt, R. B., Chader, G. J. and Gery, I. (1987). Uveitis induced in primates by IRBP: humoral and cellular immune responses. *Exp. Eye Res.*, **45**, 695–702

17. Faure, J. P., Phuc, L. H., Takano, S., Sterkers, M., Thillaye, B. and de Kozak, Y. (1981). Experimental uveoretinitis induced in monkeys by retinal S antigen. Induction, histopathology. *J. Fr. Ophtalmol.*, **4**, 465–72

18. Rodrigues, M., Hackett, J., Wiggert, B., Gery, I., Spiegel, A., Krishna, G., Stein, P. and Chader, G. (1987). Immunoelectron microscopic localization of photoreceptor-specific markers in the monkey retina. *Curr. Eye Res.*, **6**, 369–80

19. Mirshahi, M., Faure, J. P., Brisson, P., Falcon, J., Guerlotte, J. and Collin, J. (1984). S-antigen immunoreactivity in retinal rods and cones and pineal photosensitive cells. *Biol. Cell.*, **52**, 195–8

20. Pfister, C., Chabre, M., Plouet, J., Tuyen, V. V., De Kozak, Y., Faure, J. P. and Kuhn, H. (1985). Retinal S antigen identified as the 48K protein regulating light-dependent phosphodiesterase in rods. *Science*, **228**, 891–3

21. Nusenblatt, R. B., Gery, I., Ballintine, E. J. and Wacker, W. B. (1980). Cellular immune responsiveness of uveitis patients to retinal S-antigen. *Am. J. Ophthalmol.*, **89**, 173–9

22. Shinohara, T., Dietzschold, B., Craft, C. M., Wistow, G., Early, J. J., Donoso, L. A., Horwitz, J. and Tao, R. (1987). Primary and secondary structure of bovine retinal S antigen (48-kDa protein). *Proc. Natl. Acad. Sci, USA*, **84**, 6975–9

23. Yamaki, K., Tsuda, M. and Shinohara, T. (1988). The sequence of human retinal S-antigen reveals similarities with alpha-transducin. *FEBS Lett.*, **234**, 39–43

24. Tsuda, M., Syed, M., Bugra, K., Whelan, J. P., McGinnis, J. F. and Shinohara, T. (1988). Structural analysis of mouse S-antigen. *Gene*, **73**, 11–20

25. Mirshahi, M., Boucheix, C., Collenot, G., Thillaye, B. and Faure, J. P. (1985). Retinal S-antigen epitopes in vertebrate and invertebrate photoreceptors. *Invest. Ophthalmol. Vis. Sci.*, **26**, 1016–21

26. van Veen, T., Eloffson, R., Hartwing, H. G., Gery, I., Mochizuki, M., Cena, V. and Klein, D. C. (1986). Retinal S-antigen: immunocytochemical and immunochemical studies on distribution in animal photoreceptors and pineal organs. *Exp. Biol.*, **45**, 15–25

27. Gregerson, D. S., Obritsch, W. F. and Fling, S. P. (1987). Identification of a uveitogenic cyanogen bromide peptide of bovine retinal S-antigen and preparation of a uveitogenic, peptide-specific T cell line. *Eur. J. Immunol.*, **17**, 405–11

28. Stein, P. C. (1984). Experimental autoimmune uveitis induced by protease digests of bovine S-antigen in Lewis rats. *Invest. Ophthalmol. Vis. Sci. (suppl.)*, **25**, 30.

29. Donoso, L. A., Merryman, C. F., Shinohara, T., Dietzschold, B., Wistow, G., Craft, C., Morley, W. and Henry, R. T. (1986). S-antigen: identification of the MAbA9-C6 monoclonal antibody binding site and the uveitopathogenic sites. *Curr. Eye Res.*, **5**, 995–1004

30. Singh, V. K., Nussenblatt, R. B., Donoso, L. A., Yamaki, K., Chan, C. C. and Shinohara, T. (1988). Identification of a uveitopathogenic and lymphocyte proliferation site in bovine S-antigen. *Cell. Immunol.*, **115**, 413–19

31. Donoso, L. A., Merryman, C. F., Sery, T. W., Shinohara, T., Dietzschold, B., Smith, A. and Kalsow, C. M. (1987). S-antigen: characterization of a pathogenic epitope which mediates experimental autoimmune uveitis and pinealitis in Lewis rats. *Curr. Eye Res.*, **6**, 1151–9

32. Singh, V. K., Yamaki, K., Donoso, L. A. and Shinohara, T. (1988). S-antigen: experimental autoimmune uveitis induced in guinea pigs with two synthetic peptides. *Curr. Eye Res.*, **7**, 87–92

33. Donoso, L. A., Yamaki, K., Merryman, C. F., Shinohara, T., Yue, S. and Sery, T. W. (1988). Human S-antigen: characterization of uveitopathogenic sites. *Curr. Eye Res.*, **7**, 1077–85

34. Gregerson, D. S., Obritsch, W. F., Fling, S. P. and Cameron, J. D. (1986). S-antigen-specific rat T cell lines recognize peptide fragments of S-antigen and mediate experimental autoimmune uveoretinitis and pinealitis. *J. Immunol.*, **136**, 2875–82

35. Lai, Y. L., Wiggert, B., Liu, Y. P. and Chader, G. J. (1982). Interphotoreceptor retinol-binding proteins: possible transport vehicles between compartments of the retina. *Nature*, **298**, 848–9

79

36. Pfeffer, B., Wiggert, B., Lee, L., Zonnenberg, B., Newsome, D. and Chader, G. (1983). The presence of a soluble interphotoreceptor retinol-binding protein (IRBP) in the retinal interphotoreceptor space. *J. Cell Physiol.*, **117**, 333–41

37. Redmond, T. M., Wiggert, B., Robey, F. A. and Chader, G. J. (1986). Interspecies conservation of structure of interphotoreceptor reinoid-binding protein. Similarities and differences as adjudged by peptide mapping and N-terminal sequencing. *Biochem. J.*, **240**, 19–26

38. Wiggert, B., Lee, L., Rodrigues, M., Hess, H., Redmond, T. M. and Chader, G. J. (1986). Immunochemical distribution of interphotoreceptor retinoid-binding protein in selected species. *Invest. Ophthalmol. Vis. Sci.*, **27**, 1041–9

39. Rodrigues, M. M., Hackett, J., Gaskins, R., Wiggert, B., Lee, L., Redmond, M. and Chader, G. J. (1986). Interphotoreceptor retinoid-binding protein in retinal rod cells and pineal gland. *Invest. Ophthalmol. Vis. Sci.*, **27**, 844–50

40. Wiggert, B. and Chader, G. J. (1985). Monkey interphotoreceptor retinoid-binding protein (IRBP): isolation, characterization and synthesis. In Bridges, C. D. and Adler, A. J. (eds.) *The Interphotoreceptor Matrix in Health and Disease*, pp. 89–110. (New York: Alan R. Liss)

41. Fox, G. M., Kuwabara, T., Wiggert, B., Redmond, T. M., Hess, H. H., Chader, G. J. and Gery, I. (1987). Experimental autoimmune uveoretinitis (EAU) induced by retinal interphotoreceptor retinoid-binding protein (IRBP): differences between EAU induced by IRBP and by S-antigen. *Clin. Immunol. Immunopathol.*, **43**, 256–64

42. Chan, C. C., Nussenblatt, R. B., Wiggert, B., Redmond, T. M., Fujikawa, L. S., Chader, G. J. and Gery, I. (1987). Immunohistochemical analysis of experimental autoimmune uveoretinitis (EAU) induced by interphotoreceptor retinoid-binding protein (IRBP) in the rat. *Immunol. Invest.*, **16**, 63–74

43. Broekhuyse, R. M., Winkens, H. J. and Kuhlmann, E. D. (1986). Induction of experimental autoimmune uveoretinitis and pinealitis by IRBP. Comparison to uveoretinitis induced by S-antigen and opsin. *Curr. Eye Res.*, **51**, 231–40

44. Vistica, B. P., Usui, M., Kuwabara, T., Wiggert, B., Lee, L., Redmond, T. M., Chader, G. J. and Gery, I. (1987). IRBP from bovine retina is poorly uveitogenic in guinea pigs and is identical to A-antigen. *Curr. Eye Res.*, **6**, 409–17

45. Redmond, T. M., Sanui, H., Nickerson, J. M., Borst, D. E., Wiggert, B., Kuwabara, T. and Gery, I. (1988). Cyanogen bromide fragments of bovine interphotoreceptor retinoid-binding protein induce experimental autoimmune uveoretinitis in Lewis rats. *Curr. Eye Res.*, **7**, 375–85

46. Sanui, H., Redmond, T. M., Hu, L. H., Kuwabara, T., Margalit, H., Cornette, J. W., Wiggert, B., Chader, G. J. and Gery, I. (1988). Synthetic peptides derived from IRBP induce EAU and EAP in Lewis rats. *Curr. Eye Res.*, **7**, 727–35

47. Hu, L.-H., Wiggert, B., Caspi, R., Redmond, T. M., Kotake, S., Sanui, H., Chader, G. J. and Gery, I. (1989). Different epitopes of IRBP are immunodominant and immunopathogenic in different strains of rats and mice. *Invest. Ophthalmol. Vis. Sci.*, **30** (suppl.) 82

48. Donoso, L. A., Merryman, C. F., Sery, T. W., Vrabec, T., Arbizo, V. and Fong, S.-L. (1988). Human IRBP: Characterization of uveitopathogenic sites. *Curr. Eye Res.*, **7**, 1087–93

49. Marak, G. E. Jr., Shichi, H., Rao, N. A. and Wacker, W. B. (1980). Patterns of experimental allergic uveitis induced by rhodopsin and retinal rod outer segments. *Ophthalmic Res.*, **12**, 165–76

50. Meyers-Elliot, R. A., Gammon, R. A., Somner, H. L. and Shimizu, I. (1983). Experimental retinal autoimmunity (ERA) in strain 13 guinea-pigs: Induction of ERA retinopathy with rhodopsin. *Clin. Immunol. Immunopathol.*, **27**, 81–95

51. Broekhuyse, R. M., Winkens, H. J., Kuhlmann, E. D. and van Vugt, A. H. (1984). Opsin-induced experimental autoimmune retinitis in rats. *Curr. Eye Res.*, **3**, 1405–12

52. Broekhuyse, R. M., Kuhlmann, E. D., van Vugt, A. H. and Winkens, H. J. (1987). Immunological and immunopathological aspects of opsin-induced uveoretinitis. *Graefes Arch. Clin. Exp. Ophthalmol.*, **225**, 45–9

53. Schalken, J. J., Winkens, H. J., van Vugh, A. H., Bovee-Geurts, P. H., de Grip, W. J. and Broekhuyse, R. M. (1988). Rhodopsin-induced experimental autoimmune uveoretinitis: dose-dependent clinicopathological features. *Exp. Eye Res.*, **47**, 135–45

54. Quinby, P. M. and Wacker, W. B. (1967). Investigations of the mechanism of tissue damage in autoallergic uveitis. *Tex. Rep. Biol. Med.*, **25**, 493–7
55 Aronson, S. B. and McMaster, P. R. B. (1971). Passive transfer of experimental allergic uveitis. *Arch. Ophthalmol.*, **86**, 557–63
56. Mochizuki, M., Kuwabara, T., McAllister, C., Nussenblatt, R. B. and Gery, I. (1985). Adoptive transfer of experimental autoimmune uveoretinitis in rats. Immunopathogenic mechanisms and histologic features. *Invest. Ophthalmol. Vis. Sci.*, **26**, 1–9
57. Rozenszajn, L. A., Muellenberg-Coulombre, C., Gery, I., El-Saied, M., Kuwabara, T., Mochizuki, M., Lando, Z. and Nussenblatt, R. B. (1986). Induction of experimental autoimmune uveoretinitis by T cell lines. *Immunology*, **57**, 559–65
58. Caspi, R. R., Roberge, F. G., McAllister, C. G., El-Saied, M., Kuwabara, T., Gery, I., Hanna, E. and Nussenblatt, R. B. (1986). T cell lines mediating experimental autoimmune uveoretinitis (EAU) in the rat. *J. Immunol.*, **136**, 928–33
59. Lightman, S. L., Caspi, R. R., Nussenblatt, R. B. and Palestine, A. G. (1987). Antigen-directed retention of an autoimmune T cell line. *Cell. Immunol.*, **110**, 28–34
60. Chan, C. C., Caspi, R. R., Roberge, F. G. and Nussenblatt, R. B. (1988). Dynamics of experimental autoimmune uveoretinitis induced by adoptive transfer of S-antigen-specific T cell line. *Invest. Ophthalmol. Vis. Sci.*, **29**, 411–18
61. Kim, M. K., Caspi, R. R., Nussenblatt, R. B., Kuwabara, T. and Palestine, A. G. (1988). Intraocular trafficking of lymphocytes in locally induced experimental autoimmune uveoretinitis (EAU). *Cell. Immunol.*, **112**, 430–6
62. Salinas-Carmona, M. C., Nussenblatt, R. B. and Gery, I. (1982). Experimental autoimmune uveitis in the athymic nude rat. *Eur. J. Immunol.*, **12**, 480–4
63. Caspi, R. R. (1986). A rapid one-step multiwell tray test for release of soluble mediators. *J. Immunol. Meth.*, **93**, 141–4
64. Naparstek, Y., Cohen, I. R., Fuks, Z. and Vlodavsky, I. (1984). Activated T lymphocytes produce a matrix-degrading heparan sulphate endoglycosidase. *Nature*, **19**, 241–4
65. Lightman, S. (1988). Immune mechanisms in autoimmune ocular disease. *Eye*, **2**, 260–6
66. Bottazzo, G. F., Borell-Pujol, R., Hanafusa, T. and Feldman, M. (1983). Role of aberrant HLA-DR expression and antigen presentation in induction of endocrine autoimmunity. *Lancet*, **2**, 1115–19
67. Bottazzo, G. F., Todd, I., Mirakian, R. and Borrell-Pujol, R. (1986). Organ-specific autoimmunity: a 1986 overview. *Immunol. Rev.*, **94**, 137–69
68. Fontana, A. and Fierz, W. (1985). The endothelium-astrocyte immune control system of the brain. *Springer Semin. Immunopathol.*, **8**, 57–70
69. Rao, N. A., Romero, J. L., Fernandez, M. A., Sevanian, A. and Marak, G. E. Jr (1986). Effect of iron chelation on severity of ocular inflammation in an animal model. *Arch. Ophthalmol.*, **104**, 1369–71
70. Rao, N. A., Sevanian, A., Fernandez, M. A., Romero, J. L., Faure, J. P., de Kozak, Y., Till, G. O. and Marak, G. E. Jr (1987). Role of oxygen radicals in experimental allergic uveitis. *Invest. Ophthalmol. Vis. Sci.*, **28**, 886–925
71. Fujikawa, L. S., Chan, C. C., McAllister, C., Gery, I., Hooks, J. J., Detrick, B. and Nussenblatt, R. B. (1987). Retinal vascular endothelium expresses fibronectin and class II histocompatibility complex antigens in experimental autoimmune uveitis. *Cell. Immunol.*, **106**, 139–50
72. Chan, C. C., Hooks, J. J., Nussenblatt, R. B. and Detrick, B. (1986). Expressions of Ia antigen on retinal pigment epithelium in experimental autoimmune uveoretinitis. *Curr. Eye Res.*, **5**, 325–30
73. Nussenblatt, R. B., Rodrigues, M. M., Wacker, W. B., Cevario, S. J., Salinas-Carmona, M. C. and Gery, I. (1981). Clyclosporin A. Inhibition of experimental autoimmune uveitis in Lewis rats. *J. Clin. Invest.*, **67**, 1228–31
74. Marak, G. E. Jr, Wacker, W. B., Rao, N. A., Jack, R. and Ward, P. A. (1979). Effects of complement depletion on experimental allergic uveitis. *Ophthalmic Res.*, **11**, 97–107
75. McMaster, P. R., Wong, V. G. and Owens, J. D. (1976). The propensity of different guinea pigs to develop experimental autoimmune uveitis. *Mod. Probl. Ophthalmol.*, **16**, 62–71
76. De Kozak, Y., Yuan, W. S., Bogossian, M. and Faure, J. P. (1976). Humoral and cellular immunity to retinal antigens in guinea pigs. *Mod. Probl. Ophthalmol.*, **16**, 51–8
77. De Kozak, Y., Sainte-Laudy, J., Benveniste, J. and Faure, J. P. (1981). Evidence for

immediate hypersensitivity phenomena in experimental autoimmune uveoretinitis. *Eur. J. Immunol.*, **11**, 612–17

78. Mochizuki, M., Kuwabara, T., Chan, C. C., Nussenblatt, R. B., Metcalfe, D. D. and Gery, I. (1984). An association between susceptibility to experimental autoimmune uveitis and choroidal mast cell numbers. *J. Immunol.*, **133**, 1699–701

79. De Kozak, Y., Sakai, J., Sainte-Laudy, J., Faure, J. P. and Benveniste, J. (1983). Pharmacological modulation of IgE-dependent mast cell degranulation in experimental autoimmune uveoretinitis. *Jpn. J. Ophthalmol.*, **27**, 598–608

80. De Kozak, Y., Mirshahi, M., Boucheix, C. and Faure, J. P. (1987). Prevention of experimental autoimmune uveoretinitis by active immunization with autoantigen-specific monoclonal antibodies. *Eur. J. Immunol.*, **17**, 541–7

81. Jerne, N. K. (1974). Towards a network theory of the immune system. *Ann. Immunol. (Paris)*, **125C**, 373–89

82. Sharpe, A. H., Gaulton, G. N., McDade, K. K., Fields, B. N. and Greene, M. I. (1984). Syngeneic monoclonal antiidiotype can induce cellular immunity to reovirus. *J. Exp. Med.*, **160**, 1195–205

83. Lider, O., Reshef, T., Beraud, E., Ben-Nun, A. and Cohen, I. R. (1988). Anti-idiotypic network induced by T cell vaccination against experimental autoimmune encephalomyelitis. *Science*, **239**, 181–5

84. Caspi, R. R., Kuwabara, T. and Nussenblatt, R. B. (1988). Characterization of a suppressor cell line which downgrades experimental autoimmune uveoretinitis in the rat. *J. Immunol.*, **140**, 2579–84

85. Chan, C. C., Mochizuki, M., Palestine, A. G., BenEzra, D., Gery, I. and Nusenblatt, R. B. (1985). Kinetics of T lymphocyte subsets in the eyes of Lewis rats with experimental autoimmune uveitis. *Cell. Immunol.*, **96**, 430–4

86. Chan, C. C., Mochizuki, M., Nussenblatt, R. B., Palestine, A. G., McAllister, C., Gery, I. and BenEzra, D. (1985). T lymphocyte subsets in experimental autoimmune uveitis. *Clin. Immunol. Immunopathol.*, **35**, 103–10

87. Chan, C. C., Nussenblatt, R. B., Wiggert, B., Redmond, T. M., Fujikawa, L. S., Chader, G. J. and Gery, I. (1987). Immunohistochemical analysis of experimental autoimmune uveoretinitis (EAU) induced by interphotoreceptor retinoid-binding protein (IRBP) in the rat. *Immunol. Invest.*, **16**, 63–74

88. Fujino, Y., Okumura, A., Nussenblatt, R. B., Gerry, I. and Mochizuki, M. (1988). Cyclosporine-induced specific unresponsiveness to retinal soluble antigen in experimental autoimmune uveoretinitis. *Clin. Immunol. Immunopathol.*, **46**, 234–48

89. Streilein, W. J. and Niederkorn, J. Y. (1985). Characterization of the suppressor cell(s) responsible for anterior chamber-associated immune deviation (ACAID) induced in Balb/c mice by P815 cells. *J. Immunol.*, **134**, 1381–7

90. Jayaraman, S. and Bellone, C. J. (1986). Interaction of idiotype-specific T suppressor factor with the hapten-specific third-order T suppressor subset results in antigen-nonspecific suppression. *Cell. Immunol.*, **101**, 72–81

91. Roberge, F. G., Caspi, R. R., Chan, C.-C., Kuwabara, T. and Nussenblatt, R. B. (1985). Long-term culture of Müller cells from adult rats in the presence of activated lymphocytes/monocytes products. *Curr. Eye Res.*, **4**, 975–81

92. Caspi, R. R., Roberge, F. G. and Nussenblatt, R. B. (1987). Organ-resident, nonlymphoid cells suppress proliferation of autoimmune T lymphocytes. *Science*, **237**, 1029–32

93. Roberge, F. G., Caspi, R. R. and Nussenblatt, R. B. (1988). Glial retinal Müller cells produce IL-1 activity and have a dual effect on autoimmune T-helper lymphocytes. Antigen presentation manifested after removal of suppressive activity. *J. Immunol.*, **140**, 2193–6

94. Rose, N. R., Bigazzi, P. E. and Warner, N. L. (1978). *Genetic Control of Autoimmune Disease* (New York: Elsevier/North Holland.)

95. Nussenblatt, R. B. (1980). HLA and ocular disease. In Steinberg, G. M., Gery, I. and Nusenblatt, R. B. (eds.) *Immunology of the Eye, Workshop 1: Immunogenetics and Transplantation Immunity*, pp. 25–42. Washington D.C.: Information Retrieval.

96. Nepom, G. T. (1988). Immunogenetics of HLA-associated diseases. *Concepts Immunopathol.*, **5**, 80–105

97. Nussenblatt, R. B., Mittal, K. K., Ryan, S., Green, W. R. and Maumenee, A. E., (1982). Birdshot retinochoroidopathy associated with HLA-A29 and immune responsiveness to

SAg. *Am. J. Ophthalmol.*, **94**, 147–58
98. Linthicum, D. S. and Freilinger, J. A. (1982). Acute autoimmune encephalomyelitis in mice. II. Susceptibility is controlled by the combination of H-2 and histamine sensitization genes. *J. Exp. Med.*, **155**, 31–40
99. Waxman, F. J., Perryman, L. E., Hinfichs, K. J. and Coe, J. E. (1981). Genetic resistance to the induction of experimental allergic encephalomyelitis in Lewis rats. I. Genetic analysis of an apparent mutant strain with phenotypic resistance to experimental allergic encephalomyelitis. *J. Exp. Med.*, **153**, 61–74
100. Gasser, D. L., Hickey, W. F. and Gonatas, N. K. (1983). The genes for non-susceptibility to EAE in the Le-R and BH rat strains are not linked to RT1. *Immunogenetics*, **17**, 441–4
101. Linthicum, D. S., Munoz, J. J. and Blaskett, A. (1982). Acute experimental encephalomyelitis in mice. I. Adjuvant action of Bordetella pertussis is due to vasoactive amine sensitization and increased vascular permeability of the central nervous system. *Cell. Immunol.*, **73**, 229–310
102. Wilder, R. L., Allen, J. B. and Hansen, C. (1987). Thymus-dependent and -independent regulation of Ia antigen expression in situ by cells in the synovium of rats with streptococcalcell wall-induced arthritis. Differences in site and intensity of expression in euthymic, athymic, and cyclosporin A-treated LEW and F344 rats. *J. Clin. Invest.*, **79**, 1160–71
103. Caspi, R. R., Wilder, R. L., Roberge, F. G., Chan, C. C., Leake, W. C., Hansen, C. T. and Nussenblatt, R. B. (1989). Studies of EAU induction in different rat strains histocompatible in RT1. *Invest. Ophthalmol. Vis. Sci.*, **30** (Suppl.) 81
104. Nussenblatt, R. B., Palestine, A. G., Chan, C. C., Leake, W. C., Rook, A. H., Scher, I. and Gery, I. (1983). Cyclosporine therapy in the treatment of uveitis. *Transpl. Proc.*, **4** (Suppl. 1), 2914–16
105. Nussenblatt, R. B., Palestine, A. G. and Chan, C. C. (1983). Cyclosporin therapy in the treatment of intraocular inflammatory disease resistant to systemic corticosteroids and cytotoxic agents. *Am. J. Ophthalmol.*, **96**, 275–82
106. Nussenblatt, R. B., Rodrigues, M. M., Salinas-Carmona, M. C., Gery, I., Cevario, S. and Wacker, W. (1982). Modulation of experimental autoimmune uveitis with cyclosporin A. *Arch. Ophthalmol.*, **100**, 1146–9
107. Shevach, E. M. (1985). The effects of cyclosporin on the immune system. *Ann. Rev. Immunol.*, **3**, 399–425
108. Hess, A. D., Colombani, P. M. and Esa, A. H. (1986). Cyclosporine and the immune response: basic aspects. *CRC Crit. Rev. Immunol.*, **6**, 123–49
109. Nussenblatt, R. B., Salinas-Carmona, M., Waksman, B. H. and Gery, I. (1983). Cyclosporin A: alterations of the cellular immune response in S-antigen-induced experimental autoimmune uveitis. *Int. Arch. Allergy Appl. Immunol.*, **70**, 289–94
110. Nussenblatt, R. B. and Scher, I. (1985). Effects of cyclosporine on T cell subsets in experimental autoimmune uveitis. *Invest. Ophthalmol. Vis. Sci.*, **26**, 10–14.
111. Caspi, R. R., McAllister, C. G., Gery, I. and Nussenblatt, R. B. (1988). Differential effects of cyclosporins A and G on functional activation of a T-helper lymphocyte line mediating experimental autoimmune uveoretinitis. *Cell. Immunol.*, **113**, 350–60
112. Fite, K. V., Pardue, S., Bengston, L., Hayden, D. and Smyth, J. R. Jr (1986). Effects of cyclosporine in spontaneous, posterior uveitis. *Curr. Eye Res.*, **5**, 787–96
113. Palestine, A. G., Austin, A. H. III, Barlow, J. E., Antonovych, T. T., Sabnis, S. G., Preuss, H. G. and Nussenblatt, R. B. (1986). Renal histopathologic alterations in patients treated with cyclosporine for uveitis. *N. Engl. J. Med.*, **314**, 1293–8
114. Nussenblatt, R. B., Dinning, W. J., Fujikawa, L. S., Chan, C. C. and Palestine, A. G. (1985). Local cyclosporine therapy for experimental autoimmune uveitis in rats. *Arch. Ophthalmol.*, **103**, 1559–62
115. Mochizuki, M., Nussenblatt, R. B., Kuwabara, T. and Gery, I. (1985). Effects of cyclosporine and other immunosuppressive drugs on experimental autoimmune uveoretinitis in rats. *Invest. Ophthalmol. Vis. Sci.*, **26**, 226–32
116. Striph, G., Doft, B., Rabin, B. and Johnson, B. (1986). Retina S antigen-induced uveitis. The efficacy of cyclosporine and corticosteroids in treatment. *Arch. Ophthalmol.*, **104**, 114–17
117. Skolik, S. A., Palestine, A. G., Blaese, R. M., Nussenblatt, R. B. and Hess, R. A. (1988).

Treatment of experimental autoimmune uveitis in the rat with systemic succinylacetone. *Clin. Immunol. Immunopathol.*, **49**, 63–71

118. Stanford, M. R., Atkinson, E., Kasp, E. and Dumonde, D. C. (1987). Modulation of experimental retinal vasculitis using dexamethasone, cyclosporin A, and prazosin. *Eye*, **1**, 626–31

119. Kawashima, H., Fujino, Y. and Mochizuki, M. (1988). Effects of a new immunosuppressive agent, FK506, on experimental autoimmune uveoretinitis in rats. *Invest. Ophthalmol. Vis. Sci.*, **29**, 1265–71

120. Nussenblatt, R. B., Caspi, R. R., Dinning, W. J., Palestine, A. G., Hiestand, P. and Borel, J. (1986). A comparison of the effectiveness of cyclosporine A, D, and G in the treatment of experimental autoimmune uveitis in rats. *J. Immunopharmacol.*, **8**, 427–35

121. Palestine, A. G., Muellenberg-Coulombre, C. G., Kim, M. K., Gelato, M. C. and Nussenblatt, R. B. (1987). Bromocriptine and low dose cyclosporine in the treatment of experimental autoimmune uveitis in the rat. *J. Clin. Invest.*, **79**, 1078–81

122. Russell, D. H., Kibler, R., Matrisian, L., Larson, D. F., Poulos, B. and Magun, B. E. (1985). Prolactin receptors on human T and B lymphocytes: antagonism of prolactin binding by cyclosporine. *J. Immunol.*, **134**, 3027–31

123. Palestine, A. G., Nussenblatt, R. B. and Gelato, M. (1988). Therapy for human auto-immune uveitis with low-dose cyclosporine plus bromocriptine. *Transplant. Proc.*, **20** (Suppl. 4), 131–5

124. Sriram, S. and Steinman, L. (1983). Anti I-A antibody suppresses active encephalomyelitis: treatment model for diseases linked to IR genes. *J. Exp. Med.*, **158**, 1362–7

125. Wetzig, R., Hooks, J. J., Percopo, C. M., Nussenblatt, R. B., Chan, C. C. and Dertick, B. (1988). Anti-Ia antibody diminishes ocular inflammation in experimental autoimmune uveitis. *Curr. Eye Res.*, **7**, 809–18

126. Osawa, H. and Diamantstein, T. (1983). The characteristics of a monoclonal antibody that binds specifically to rat T lymphoblasts and inhibits IL 2 receptor functions. *J. Immunol.*, **130**, 51–5

127. Higuchi, M., Nussenblatt, R. B., Diamantstein, T., Osawa, H. and Caspi, R. R. (1989). Combined anti-interleukin-2 receptor and low-dose cyclosporin therapy in experimental autoimmune uveoretinitis. *Invest. Ophthalmol. Vis. Sci.* **30** (Suppl.) 85

128. Roberge, F. G., LeHoang, P., Chan, C. C., Nussenblatt, R. B., Pastan, I. and Lorberboum-Galski, H. (1989). Treatment of experimental autoimmune uveoretinitis with IL2-PE40, a T cell targeted chimeric toxin. *Invest. Ophthalmol. Vis. Sci.*, **30** (Suppl.) 279

129. Lorberboum-Galski, H., FitzGerald, D., Chaudhary, V., Adhya, S. and Pastan, I. (1988). Cytotoxic activity of an interleukin 2-Pseudomonas exotoxin chimeric protein produced in Escherichia coli. *Proc. Natl. Acad. Sci. USA*, **85**, 1922–6

130. Cohen, I. R. (1986). Regulation of autoimmune disease physiological and therapeutic. *Immunol. Rev.*, **94**, 5–21

131. Lider, O., Karin, N., Shinitzky, M. and Cohen, I. R. (1987). Therapeutic vaccination against adjuvant arthritis using autoimmune T cells treated with hydrostatic pressure. *Proc. Natl. Acad. Sci. USA*, **84**, 4577–80

132. Lamont, A. G., Bruce, M. G., Watret, K. C. and Ferguson, A. (1988). Suppression of an established DTH response to ovalbumin in mice by feeding antigen after immunization. *Immunology*, **64**, 135–9

133. Gautam, S. C. and Battisto, J. R. (1985). Orally induced tolerance generates an efferently acting suppressor T cell and an acceptor T cell that together down-regulate contact sensitivity. *J. Immunol.*, **135**, 2975–83

134. Silverman, G. A., Peri, B. A., Fitch, F. W. and Rothberg, R. M. (1983). Enterically induced regulation of systemic immune responses. II. Suppression of proliferating T cells by an Lyt-1+, 2-T effector cell. *J. Immunol.*, **131**, 2656–61

135. Mattingly, J. A. and Waksma, B. H. (1978). Immunologic suppression after oral admin-istration of antigen. I. Specific suppressor cells formed in rat Peyer's patches after oral administration of sheep erythrocytes and their systemic migration. *J. Immunol.*, **121**, 1878–1883

136. Higgins, P. J. and Weiner, H. L. (1988). Suppression of experimental autoimmune encephalomyelitis by oral administration of myelin basic protein and its fragments. *J. Immunol.*, **140**, 440–5

137. Bitar, D. M. and Whitacre, C. C. (1988). Suppression of experimental autoimmune encephalomyelitis by the oral administration of myelin basic protein. *Cell. Immunol.*, **112**, 364–70

138. Rosenbaum, J. T., McDevitt, H. O., Guss, R. B. and Egbert, P. R. (1980). Endotoxin-induced uveitis in rats as a model for human disease. *Nature*, **286**, 611–13

139. Levene, R. Z. and Breinin, G. M. (1959). Ocular effects of endotoxin. *Arch. Ophthalmol.*, **61**, 113–25

140. Cousins, S. W., Guss, R. B., Howes, E. L. Jr and Rosenbaum, J. T. (1984). Endotoxin-induced uveitis in the rat: observations of altered vascular permeability, clinical findings, and histology. *Exp. Eye Res.*, **39**, 665–76

141. Howes, E. L. Jr, Hartiala, K. T., Webster, R. O. and Rosenbaum, J. T. (1985). Complement and polymorphonuclear leukocytes do not determine the vascular permeability induced by intraocular LPS. *Am. J. Pathol.*, **118**, 35–42

142. Bhattacherjee, P. (1975). Release of prostaglandin-like substances by Shigella endotoxin and its inhibition by non-steroidal anti-inflammatory compounds. *Br. J. Pharmacol.*, **54**, 489–94

143. Rosenbaum, J. T., Raymond, W., Seymour, B. W., Wolfrom, J. A., Enkel, H. and Howes, E. L. Jr (1986). The effect of corticosteroids or nitrogen mustard on aqueous humor chemotactic activity induced by intravitreal endotoxin. *Clin. Immunol. Immunopathol.*, **39**, 414–20

144. Rosenbaum, J. T., Langlois, L., Enkel, H. and Wolfrom, J. A. (1985). Modification of lipid A reduces endotoxin-induced eye effects. *Curr. Eye Res.*, **4**, 707–11

145. Fleisher, L. N. (1988). Effects of inhibitors of arachidonic acid metabolism on endotoxin-induced ocular inflammation. *Curr. Eye Res.*, **7**, 321–327

146. Kim, M. K., Palestine, A. G., Nussenblatt, R. B. and Chan, C. C. (1986). Expression of Class II antigen in endotoxin induced uveitis. *Curr. Eye Res.*, **5**, 869–76

147. Howes, E. L. Jr and Morrison, D. C. (1980). Lipid A dependence of the ocular response to circulating endotoxin in rabbits. *Infect. Immun.*, **30**, 786–90

148. Rosenbaum, J. J., Howes, E. L. Jr, Rubin, R. M. and Samples. J. R. (1988). Ocular inflammatory effects of intravitreally-injected tumor necrosis factor. *Am. J. Pathol.*, **133**, 47–53

149. Rosenbaum, J. T., Hendricks, P. A., Shively, J. E. and McDougall, I. R. (1983). Distribution of radiolabelled endotoxin with particular reference to the eye: concise communication. *J. Nucl. Med.*, **24**, 29–33

150. Howes, E. L. Jr, Hoffman, M. A., Ulevitch, R. J., Mathison, J. C. and Morrison, D. C. (1984). Ocular localization of circulating bacterial lipopolysaccharide. *Exp. Eye Res.*, **38**, 379–89

151. Wells, A., Pararajasegaram, G., Baldwin, M., Yang, C. H., Hammer, M. and Fox, A. (1986). Uveitis and arthritis induced by systemic injection of streptococcal cell walls. *Invest. Ophthalmol. Vis. Sci.*, **27**, 921–5

152. Howes, E. L. Jr, Char, D. H. and Christensen, M. (1982) Aqueous immune complexes in immunogenic uveitis. *Invest. Ophthalmol. Vis. Sci.*, **23**, 715–18

153. Lightman, S., Palestine, A. and Nussenblatt, R. (1986). Immunohistopathology of experimental uveitis induced by a non-ocular antigen. *Curr. Eye Res.*, **5**, 857–62

154. Donnelly, J. J. and Prendergast, R. A. (1984). Local production of Ia-inducing activity in experimental immunogenic uveitis. *Cell. Immunol.*, **86**, 557–61

155. Sher, N. A., Foon, K. A., Fishman, M. L. and Brown, T. M. (1976). Demonstration of macrophage chemotactic factors in the aqueous humour during experimental immunogenic uveitis in rabbits. *Infect. Immun.*, **13**, 1110–16

156. Rosenbaum, J. T., Seymour, B. W., Raymond, W., Langlois, L., Wu, M. and David, L. (1988). Similar chemotactic factor for monocytes predominates in different animal models of uveitis. *Inflammation*, **12**, 191–201

157. Kulkarni, P. S., Bhattacherjee, P., Eakins, K. E. and Srinivasan, B. D. (1981). Anti-inflammatory effects of betamethasone phosphate, dexamethasone phosphate and indomethacin on rabbit ocular inflammation induced by bovine serum albumin. *Curr. Eye Res.*, **1**, 43–47

158. Chan, C. C. (1988). Relationship between sympathetic ophthalmia, phacoanaphylatic endophthalmitis, and Vogt-Kayanagi-Harada disease. *Ophthalmology*, **95**, 619–24

159. Marak, G. E. Jr, Rao, N. A., Antonakou, G. and Sliwinski, A. (1982). Experimental lens-induced granulomatous endophthalmitis in common laboratory animals. *Ophthalmic Res.*, **14**, 292–7

160. Kraus-Mackiw, E., Buttner, K. and Müller-Ruchholtz, W. M. (1977). Lens-induced uveitis: further immunological studies in an experimental model. *Graefes Arch. Clin. Exp. Ophthalmol.*, **202**, 297–303

161. Rao, N. A., Calandra, A. J., Sevanian, A., Bowe, B., Delmage, J. M. and Marak, G. E. Jr (1986). Modulation of lens-induced uveitis by superoxide dismutase. *Ophthal. Res.*, **18**, 41–6

162. Rao, N. A., Fernandez, M. A., Sevanian, A., Romero, J. L., Till, G. O. and Marak, G. E. Jr (1988). Treatment of experimental lens-induced uveitis by dimethyl thiourea. *Opthal. Res.*, **20**, 106–11

163 Rao, N. A., Patchett, R., Fernandez, M. A., Sevanian, A., Kunkel, S. L. and Marak, G. E. Jr (1987). Treatment of experimental granulomatous uveitis by lipoxygenase and cyclo-oxygenase inhibitors. *Arch Ophthalmol.*, **105**, 413–25

164. Lang, R. A., Metcalf, D., Cuthbertson, R. A., Lyons, I., Stanley, E., Kelso, A., Kannourakis, G., Williamson, D. J., Klintworth, G. K. and Gonda, T. J. (1987). Transgenic mice expressing a hemopoietic growth factor gene (GM-CSF) develop accumulations of macrophages, blindness, and a fatal syndrome of tissue damage. *Cell*, **51**, 675–86

6
Immunopathology of Ocular Inflammatory Disorders

S. LIGHTMAN and C.-C. CHAN

INTRODUCTION

Ocular inflammation can occur in patients with systemic disorders such as sarcoidosis and Behçet's disease or can be localized to the eyes as in sympathetic ophthalmia and pars planitis. Many of these disorders have characteristic features that are recognizable clinically but whose causes are unknown. The patient often requires immunosuppressive therapy to control the inflammatory response so as to limit the damage to the ocular tissue. Autoimmune mechanisms are thought to be involved in the initiation and/or perpetuation of the inflammatory response, although the exact role in the pathogenesis is unknown. With the advent of immunohistochemical staining with monoclonal antibodies to cell surface markers, much more is now known about the cell types infiltrating the inflamed eyes in these conditions.

Many of the inflamed eyes that have been examined immunohistopathologically have been enucleated at the end-stages of the disease processes, after the development of complications and/or after systemic immunosuppressive therapy. The findings are therefore of one time point and may reflect different pathology from that seen in the acute phase of the disease. With that proviso in mind, the findings in several clinically recognized ocular inflammatory states will be presented and discussed.

SYMPATHETIC OPHTHALMIA

Sympathetic ophthalmia (SO) has been known about since the time of Hippocrates and the initiating factors are still not known. It is defined as a bilateral inflammation of the entire uveal tract that follows perforating injury to one eye, either in the form of trauma from a penetrating injury or following intraocular surgery. In 90% of cases, the inflammation occurs within 1 year of the injury, with 65% occurring within the first 2 months[1]. More uncommonly,

87

many years may elapse before the onset of the inflammatory process. Clinically, there is a bilateral panuveitis with choroidal thickening and optic nerve swelling. Dalen–Fuchs nodules characteristically occur in the periphery and appear as whitish-yellow spots at the level of the retinal pigment epithelium (RPE)[2]. The disease usually follows a relapsing course and treatment is aimed at immunosuppression, usually with steroids in the first instance but other drugs such as azathioprine, cyclophosphamide and cyclosporin may be useful[3].

Histopathologically, there is a diffuse non-necrotizing granulomatous inflammation of the uvea with marked thickening of the choroid and relative sparing of the retina and choriocapillaris, with similar appearances seen in both the injured and the sympathizing eye. The choroid is infiltrated by lymphocytes with nests of macrophages, epithelioid and giant cells. Dalen–Fuchs nodules, seen in 30–100% of cases examined depending on the series, consist mainly of epithelioid cells located between Bruch's membrane and the RPE[4].

In an American series, 32% of 28 patients with SO were found to have the HLA-A11 antigen as compared to 4% of 107 patients with ocular perforation but without SO[5]. The antigens HLA-DR4 and HLA-DRW53 were found to be highly associated with SO in Japanese patients[6]. Histological variants related to race have been reported between Black and White American patients with SO[7], but no difference was seen between Chinese and American patients[8].

Immunohistopathological studies of SO demonstrate that the choroid is infiltrated mainly by T lymphocytes with a small number of B cells and plasma cells[9–11]. In the eyes enucleated early in the disease process, the T cells were mainly of the CD4+ type[12] and of the CD8+ type in later stages (Figure 6.1). In most series, there was no alteration of the T cell populations in the patient's blood[9,11,13]. The epithelioid cells in Dalen–Fuchs nodules express Class II MHC antigens (HLA-DR) and have the staining characteristics of bone-marrow derived histiocytes[9,10,11,14]. They may be involved in presenting ocular antigens to T cells. The T cell infiltration suggests that it is the cellular rather than the humoral arm of the immune response that is predominantly activated. This was suggested previously by the demonstration of lymphocyte transformation to crude extracts of uveoretinal tissue[15] in patients with this disease.

The inciting antigen in sympathetic ophthalmia is still not known. Neither uveal melanin nor uveal homogenates are immunogenic[16], but retinal extracts, and in particular retinal S-antigen[17] and interphotoreceptor binding protein (IRBP)[18], are highly antigenic and are able to induce uveoretinitis (which can mimic several features of SO) in experimental animals[19] when given with adjuvants[20]. Exactly how relevant these antigens are in man is unknown. It is possible that penetrating trauma, however caused, may result in the exposure of uveoretinal antigens to conjunctival lymphatics[21], with infectious agents such as bacteria and viruses in genetically susceptible individuals acting as adjuvants for induction of the disease[22,23].

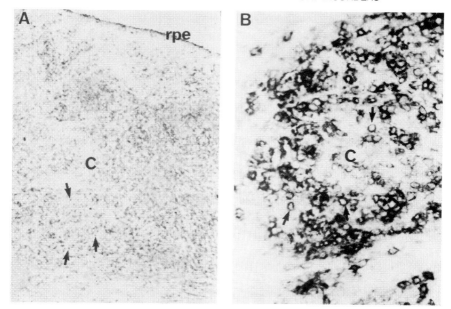

Figure 6.1 Sympathetic ophthalmia: (A) early and (B) late stages. Choroid infiltrated with T cells (arrows) of the CD4+ type (A) and CD8+ type (B). C = choroid; rpe = retinal pigment epithelium. Frozen section: (A) × 268; (B) × 536

VOGT-KOYANAGI-HARADA (VKH) SYNDROME

VKH syndrome occurs more frequently in Orientals, in whom it accounts for 8% of uveitis patients[24], but in Americans only 1–4% of uveitis patients were diagnosed as having the VKH syndrome[25]. The panuveitis may be preceded by a prodromal phase characterized by headaches, orbital pain, meningism and nausea, and examination of the CSF may show a pleocytosis. Ocular involvement is usually bilateral, although one eye may present first, and is associated with a panuveitis, optic nerve swelling, serous detachment of the retina and infiltration of both the choroid and RPE. Poliosis, vitiligo, alopecia, dysacousia may also occur. The retina reattaches with a mottled appearance and there may be chorioretinal scarring[25,26]. Systemic involvement is not associated with a worse visual prognosis[25].

In Japan, a study of 185 patients with VKH were reported to express the HLA-DRW53 antigen and there was increased expression of HLA-DR4 and HLA-DQWa as compared to controls[27]. HLA typing of 17 American patients with VKH did not reveal any strong associations[28].

Histopathological examination demonstrates many features of sympathetic ophthalmia but also obliteration of the choriocapillaris, focal active chorioretinitis and marked involvement of the RPE[29,30]. In a patient with long-standing disease, T lymphocyte infiltration was seen in the uvea and retina but, in contrast to SO, foci of aggregated B lymphocytes were also

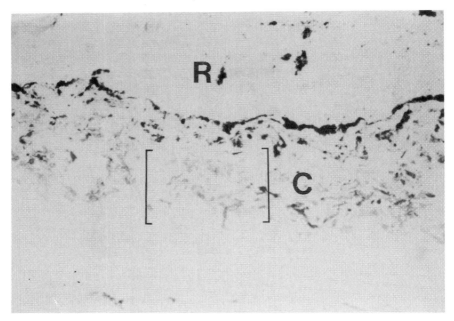

Figure 6.2 VKH syndrome. Immunohistochemical examination showed a foci (brackets) of B (CD22+) lymphocytes infiltrating the choroid. R = retina; C = choroid. Frozen section × 250

seen[31] (Figure 6.2). An increase in serum IgD has also been reported[32]. Limbal biopsies in patients with VKH demonstrated an increase in CD4+ T cells in early stages of the disease and an increase in CD8+ cells at a later stage[33]. T cells have also been found in the CSF and in skin lesions[33] and an increase in interferon-γ has been demonstrated in the serum of CSF of patients with VKH[27]. Antibodies to ganglioside[28], outer segments of the photoreceptors and Müller cells[34] have all been detected, as has evidence for cell-mediated immunity to myelin basic protein[35] and melanin[36]. It is postulated that an unknown agent such as a virus may trigger an autoimmune reaction to the melanocytes and/or neuronal elements.

PARS PLANITIS

Pars planitis, a chronic ocular inflammatory disorder, is characterized by "snowbanks" overlying the pars planna occurring particularly in children and young adults[37]. There is often optic nerve swelling and macular oedema with patchy leakage from the retinal veins demonstrable on fluorescein angiography[38]. Neovascularization may occur in the region of the snowbank which can result in preretinal membrane formation and subsequently in traction retinal detachment. No genetic linkage to HLA loci has been identified although there have been reports of the disease occurring in siblings[39].

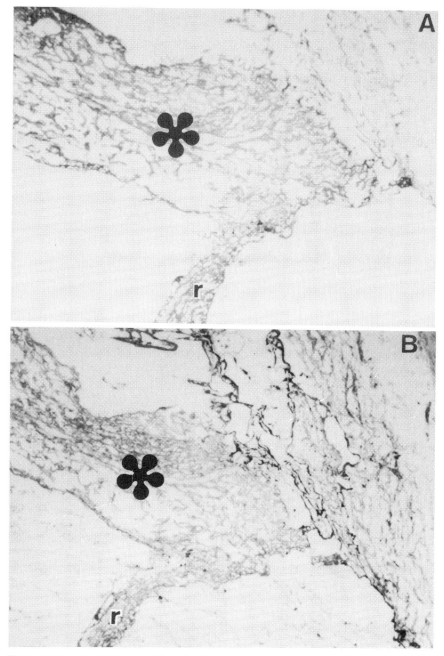

Figure 6.3 Pars planitis. Immunohistochemical examination showed the main component of the snowbank (star) staining positively for (A) GFAP and (B) Müller monoclonal antibody. r = retina. Frozen section × 100

Enucleated eyes have demonstrated detachment and collapse of the vitreous body with fibrous organization of the vitreous base[40]. Either no significant choroiditis or small focal areas of peripheral choroiditis were seen with low-grade lymphocytic infiltration of the pars plana[41]. Examination of the snowbank showed that it contained vascularized condensed vitreous collagen with interspersed chronic inflammatory cells and hyperplastic non-pigmented ciliary epithelium together with fibroglial tissue. It was suggested that the snowbank arose from a common inflammatory process involving both the peripheral retina and the vitreous base[42].

An immunohistopathological study of an eye with end-stage pars planitis demonstrated an influx of CD4+ T cells into the pars plana, snowbank and around the retinal vessels[43]. Few of the T cells had demonstrable IL-2 receptors. Normal peripheral blood T cell populations were found. B cells were seen in the iris and ciliary body but not in the snowbank or pars plana. The snowbank stained heavily with antibodies against glial fibrillary acid protein (GFAP) and Müller cells (Figure 6.3) suggesting that glial elements are involved in the snowbank. Type IV collagen and laminin were the major collagen glycoproteins in the snowbank and these are known to be formed by glial cells rather than fibroblasts[42]. This suggests that the snowbank may be formed from glial elements in the peripheral retina.

Müller cells are known to proliferate in vitro in response to factors produced by activated T cells[44], suggesting that the snowbank formation might be stimulated by the inflammatory process. These cells can also present antigens to T cells[45] in vitro and therefore might contribute themselves to the inflammatory process. Why this type of ocular inflammation stimulates a glial response, whereas it is uncommon in other types, is completely unknown.

SARCOIDOSIS

Sarcoidosis is a systemic granulomatous disorder of unknown aetiology[46]. Hilar lymphadenopathy and pulmonary infiltration are common findings, but many organ systems can become involved, including skin, joints, liver and central nervous system. In the eye there is usually an anterior uveitis, classically with mutton-fat keratic precipitates, vitritis and retinal vasculitis[47]. The retinal vessels may be sheathed and show patchy leakage of dye on fluorescein angiography. Branch vein occlusions can occur. Retinal and macular oedema may occur and retinal granulomas may extend into and involve the choroid[48,49]. The optic nerves can be involved by extension from the retinal inflammatory process, by granulomas primarily affecting the nerve itself, or from raised intracranial pressure due to CNS involvement.

In the peripheral blood, there is a generalized lymphopenia with marked reduction in the number of T-helper cells, a decreased response to mitogens and depressed B cell function[50]. Histopathologically, sarcoidosis is characterized by non-caseating granulomas mainly composed of macrophages, epithelioid cells and giant cells surrounded by a rim of lymphocytes[46]. An infiltrate of CD4+ T cells was found in the lungs, liver, skin, lymph nodes and

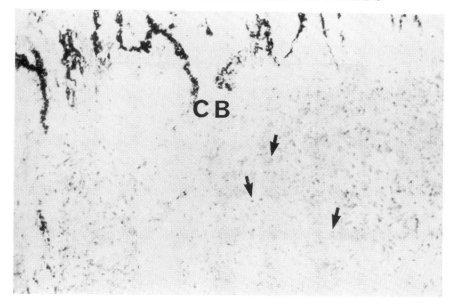

Figure 6.4 Sarcoidosis. Ciliary body infiltration with CD4+ T cells (arrows). Frozen section × 380

conjunctiva of patients with active sarcoidosis[51].

An eye enucleated from a patient with active sarcoidosis because it had become blind and painful as a result of severe intraocular inflammation was examined immunohistopathologically[52]. Within the granulomas found in the retina and uvea, 90% of the T cells were of the CD4+ phenotype (Figure 6.4). Fewer than 10% of the total T cells were CD8+ and these were confined to the lymphocyte cuff and were not within the granulomas. Lymphocytes both within and around the granuloma had demonstrable IL-2 receptors as did the epithelioid and giant cells. Class II MHC antigens were diffusely distributed over the granuloma. T cells and activated macrophages were closely associated within the granuloma and binding of anti-interferon-γ antibody was found in the granuloma. Very few B cells were seen and those were at the periphery of the granulomas. These findings suggest that the T cells seen in the granulomas are activated and secreting both IL-2 and interferon-γ. The macrophages were found to express Class II MHC antigens, suggesting that they are involved in antigen presentation to the T cells.

A ring of CD8+ cells was present surrounding the granuloma and it is tempting to think that these cells are acting to restrict the cell-mediated immune response[53,54]. The tissue findings, including those described in the eye, suggest that sarcoidosis is a disease of heightened cell-mediated immune activity in affected tissues. This results in massive recruitment of CD4+ T cells from the peripheral blood and the cutaneous anergy seen on PPD testing in patients previously immunized with BCG[55].

BEHÇET'S DISEASE

This disorder is characterized by an occlusive vasculitis and can affect many different organ systems. There are several forms of this disease, which can overlap. The type of disease with mainly ocular features is said to be associated with HLA-B51, a subtype of B5[56]. HLA-B12 is associated with the type that affects mainly the skin and mucous membranes[57]. All forms may be associated with mouth ulceration, which is a classic diagnostic feature. The ocular disease is characterized by a panuveitis and occlusive retinal vasculitis, classically with hypopyon[58]. A viral cause, particularly a herpes virus, has been implicated many times as the causative agent in Behçet's disease[59,60] but this aetiology remains unproven. However, whether the disease process is initially triggered by infection with herpes simplex or another virus is unknown.

More recently, streptococcal antigens have been found in the lesions (aphthous ulcer and skin lesion) of Behçet's disease and lymphocytes from these patients proliferated *in vitro* when cultured with the streptococcal antigen. It was suggested that in Behçet's disease, insufficient anti-streptococcal antibodies were formed so that there was not adequate neutralization of the streptococcal antigens. Other groups have found increased circulating IgA reacting to *Streptococcus pyogenes* antigen, and a significantly higher level of IgA in the circulating immune complexes in serum from patients with Behçet's disease. Although skin testing with streptococcus antigen was unhelpful, lymphocytes from patients with Behçet's disease showed a higher stimulation index to the same antigen when co-cultured *in vitro*, suggesting sensitization of the lymphocytes to this antigen[61]. The significance of these findings is uncertain. Some features of the ocular disease seen in Behçet's disease were seen in rats after immunization with polysaccharides extracted from the cell walls of *S. pyogenes*[62].

Complexes of IgG and the complement components C3 and C5 have been found in the aqueous humour[63] which are thought to be chemotactic for polymorphonuclear leukocytes. Circulating immune complexes and altered levels of C3 may be found in the serum of patients with Behçet's disease[64]. Shimada *et al.*[65] found an acute reduction in complement levels immediately prior to an attack and suggested it was being taken up by tissue-bound immune complexes. It has been shown that there is enhanced neutrophil migration as a result of immune-complex-mediated damage to the endothelial cells of the blood vessels, and *in vitro* colchicine can block the enhanced migration of lymphocytes induced by serum from Behçet's patients. This may account, in part, for the therapeutic effects of colchicine seen in some of these patients[66].

No impairment of cell-mediated immunity was detected in patients with Behçet's disease as determined by skin testing with PPD and mumps, although a decrease in total numbers of T cells has been reported. A lower T4:T8 ratio was seen in the peripheral blood in patients with one or more of the major manifestations of Behçet's disease, including uveitis. Abnormal B-cell function with increased amounts of circulating IgG, IgA, IgM, reduced natural killer cell activity and a decreased ability of their T lymphocytes to

94

produce and respond to IL-2 have also been reported[67].

Histological examination of the retina reveals numerous areas of vascular occlusion affecting both the arteries and veins. The superficial layers of the retina may undergo necrosis and there is atrophy of the nerve fibre layer secondary to the progressive ischaemia and loss of blood-supply. The affected retinal vessels show thickened basement membranes with mucopolysaccharide deposition. Thrombus is present in the vessel lumen and the area around the vessel is infiltrated with polymorphonuclear leukocytes and lymphocytes[68].

Although no eyes have to date been examined immunohistopathologically, biopsies of erythema nodosum-like skin lesions have been taken[69]. Early lesions were characterized by large numbers of infiltrating lymphocytes and macrophages, particularly in the perivascular areas; 60–80% of the lymphocytes were found to be T cells of the CD4+ type with 20–40% of the T cells being of the CD8+ type. NK cells were found in the infiltrate in 50% of biopsies examined and only constituted 5% of the total cellular infiltrate. B cells were not present. In older lesions, the pathological picture was much more varied and the infiltrate consisted mainly of neutrophils rather than lymphocytes. Similar examination of oral ulcers within 3 days of development also showed a predominance of T lymphocytes in the infiltrate, with less than 15% of the total cells being B cells. Equal numbers of CD4+ and CD8+ cells were seen in this study[70].

DISCUSSION

Although these studies give no information on the aetiology of these inflammatory disorders, they do implicate the CD4+ T cell as playing a major role in the active inflammatory lesion. Few B cells are seen in the tissues apart from in the study of the eye with VKH syndrome, but, even in this eye, T cells still greatly outnumber the B cells. Class II MHC antigens were demonstrated to be present in some resident cells of the eyes, suggesting that there is active presentation of antigen to the infiltrating T cells.

CD4+ T cells have been shown *in vitro* to be functionally heterogeneous and, recently, murine CD4+ T cells have been divided into two groups (Th$_1$ and Th$_2$) on the basis of which lymphokines they are able to secrete, because the latter determine the function of each T cell. Th$_1$ cells secrete IL-2, interferon-γ and lymphotoxin, whereas Th$_2$ cells secrete IL-4. IL-2 production is important because it has many functions, including the maturation of Class I MHC restricted cytotoxic T cells. Interferon-γ induces Class II MHC expression and thereby enhances local antigen presentation. Th$_1$ CD4+ T cells may also be cytotoxic but will only kill target cells expressing Class II MHC antigens. Lymphotoxin is thought to be one of the cytotoxic lymphokines secreted by these cells, although it is not the only one[71]. IL-4 is a B-cell maturation lymphokine and 'helps' in antibody production by B cells. The situation in man appears not so clear-cut, at least *in vitro*, as CD4+ T cell clones have been found that secrete both IL-2 and IL-4[72]. The *in vivo* situation requires further clarification and it is not known whether the CD4+ T cell is itself an effector cell or whether its main function is to recruit into the tissues other cell types that actually do the damage.

Current theories of autoimmune diseases suggest that their aetiology is likely to be a complicated mixture of genetic, immunological and viral factors. These factors may determine the site of the disease process and therefore its clinical features. If the means by which these diseases are perpetuated in the tissues can be elucidated, it may be possible in the future to pharmacologically switch off lymphokine production by these activated CD4+ cells and prevent further damage occurring. Cyclosporin is a start in that direction, as it prevents IL-2 and interferon-γ production and release. Until that time, these patients will be given intensive immunosuppressive therapy with all its accompanying problems and many will still lose their vision.

References

1. Lubin, J., Albert, D. and Weinstein, M. (1980). Sixty-five years of sympathetic ophthalmia. *Ophthalmology*, **87**, 109–21
2. Marak, G. (1979). Recent advances in sympathetic ophthalmia. *Surv. Ophthalmol.*, **24**, 141–56
3. Nussenblatt, R., Palestine, A. and Chan, C. (1983). Cyclosporine therapy in the treatment of intraocular disease resistant to systemic steroids or cytotoxic agents. *Am. J. Ophthalmol.*, **96**, 275–82
4. Green, W. (1986). Inflammatory diseases and conditions of the eye. In Spencer, W. (ed.) *Ophthalmic Pathology*, Vol III, pp. 1923–66. (Philadelphia: W. B. Saunders)
5. Reynard, M., Schulman, I., Azen, S. and Minckler, D. (1983). Histocompatibility antigens in sympathetic ophthalmia. *Am. J. Ophthalmol.*, **95**, 216–21
6. Ohno, S. (1988). Immunogenetic studies on ocular disease. In Blodi, F. *et al.* (eds.) *Acta XXV Concilium Ophthalmologicum*. Kugler and Ghedini. Proceedings of the XV International Congress of Ophthalmology, Rome, May 1986. **1**, 144–54
7. Marak, G., Font, R. and Zimmerman, L. (1974). Histologic variations related to race in sympathetic ophthalmia. *Am. J. Ophthalmol.*, **781**, 935–8
8. Kuo, P., Lubin, J., Ni, C., Wang, K. and Albert, D. (1982). Sympathetic ophthalmia. *Int. Clin. Ophthalmol.*, **22**, 125–39
9. Jakobiec, F., Marboe, C., Knowles, D., Iwamoto, T., Harrison, W., Chang, S. and Coleman, D. (1983). Human sympathetic ophthalmia. *Ophthalmology*, **90**, 76–95
10. Chan, C., BenEzra, D., Rodrigues, M., Palestine, A., Hsu, S., Murphree, A. and Nussenblatt, R. (1984). Immunohistochemistry and electron microscopy of choroidal infiltrates and Dalen–Fuchs nodules in sympathetic ophthalmia. *Ophthalmology*, **92**, 580–90
11. Chan, C., Nussenblatt, R., Fujikawa, L., Palestine, A., Stevens, G., Parver, L., Luckenbach, M. and Kuwabara, T. (1986). Sympathetic ophthalmia: immunological findings. *Ophthalmology*, **93**, 690–5
12. Müller-Hermelink, H., Kraus-Mackiv, E. and Daus, W. (1984). Early stage of human sympathetic ophthalmia. *Arch. Ophthalmol.*, **102**, 1753–7
13. Boone, W., Gupta, S., Hansen, J. and Good, R. (1976). Lymphocyte subpopulations in patients with sympathetic uveitis. *Invest. Ophthalmol. Vis. Sci.*, **15**, 957–60.
14. Rao, N., Xu, S. and Font, R. (1985). Sympathetic ophthalmia: An immunohistochemical study of epithelioid and giant cells. *Ophthalmology*, **92**, 1660–2
15. Rahi, A., Morgan, G., Levy, I. and Dinning, W. (1978). Immunological investigations in post-traumatic granulomatous and non-granulomatous uveitis. *Br. J. Ophthalmol.*, **62**, 722–8
16. Urgancioglu, M., Halpern, B., Parlebas, J. and Rebeyrotte, P. (1970). Concerning the antigenicity of the constituents of the uvea. *Rev. Immunol. (Paris)*, **34**, 85–97
17. Faure, J., DeKozak, Y., Dorey, C., Tuyen, C. and Tuyen, V. (1977). Activity of different antigenic preparations from the retina to induce experimental autoimmune uveoretinitis.

Arch. Ophthalmol. (Paris), **37**, 47–60
18. Gery, I., Mochizuki, M. and Nussenblatt, R. (1986). Retinal specific antigens and immunopathogenetic processes they provoke. In Osbourne, N. and Chader, J. (eds.) *Progress in Retinal Research* pp. 75–109. (Oxford: Pergamon Press)
19. Faure, J. (1980). Autoimmunity and the retina. *Curr. Top. Eye Res.*, **2**, 215–302
20. Marak, G. (1979). Recent advances in sympathetic ophthalmia. *Surv. Ophthalmol.*, **24**, 141–56
21. Rao, N. and Marak, G. (1983). Sympathetic ophthalmia simulating VKH disease. *Jpn. J. Ophthalmol.*, **27**, 506–11
22. Rao, N. and Cook, G. (1980). Sympathetic uveitis. *Contemp. Ophthalmol.*, **1**, 1–6
23. Rao, N. and Wong, V. (1981). Aetiology of sympathetic ophthalmitis. *Trans. Ophthalmol. Soc. U.K.*, **101**, 357–60
24. Suguira, S. (1978). Vogt–Koyanagi–Harada disease. *Jpn. J. Ophthalmol.*, **22**, 9–35
25. Ohno, S., Char, D., Kimura, S. and O'Connor, G. (1977). Vogt–Koyanagi–Harada syndrome. *Am. J. Ophthalmol.*, **83**, 735–40
26. Schimizu, K. (1973). Harada's, Behçet's, VKH syndromes – are they clinical entities? *Trans. Am. Acad. Ophthalmol. Otolaryngol.*, **77**, 281–90
27. Ohno, S (1984). Vogt–Koyanagi–Harada's disease. In Saari, K. (ed.) *Uveitis Update*, pp. 401–5. (Amsterdam: Elsevier Science Publishers.)
28. Yokoyama, M., Matsui, Y., Kamashiroya, H., O'Donell, M., Tseng, H., Stryder, D., Tessler, H., Crisfen, R. and Zimjewski, C. (1981). Humoral and cellular immunity studies in patients with VKH syndrome and pars planitis. *Invest. Ophthalmol. Vis. Sci.*, **20**, 364–70
29. Perry, H. and Font, R. (1977). Clinical and histopathologic observations in severe Vogt–Koyanagi–Harada syndrome. *Am. J. Ophthalmol.*, **83**, 242–54
30. Lubin, J., Ni, C. and Albert, D. (1982). A clinicopathological study of Vogt–Koyanagi–Harada syndrome. *Int. Ophthalmol. Clin.*, **22**, 141–56
31. Chan, C., Palestine, A., Kuwabara, T. and Nussenblatt, R. (1988). Immunopathologic study of Vogt–Koyanagi–Harada syndrome. *Am. J. Ophthalmol.*, **105**, 607–11
32. Moriyama, H., Matsumoto, K. and Mimura, Y. (1976). Serum immunoglobulin D in Harada's disease and Behçet's disease. *Acta Soc. Ophthalmol. Jpn.*, **80**, 480–5
33. Aniga, H., Ohno, S., Higuchi, M., Taniguchi, M., Nakamura, A. and Yoshiki, T. (1989). Immunological studies on lymphocytes in the CSF of patients with Vogt–Koyanagi–Harada disease. *Clin. Immunol. (Jpn)* (In press)
34. Chan, C., Nussenblatt, R., Palestine, A., Roberge, F. and BenEzra, D. (1985). Anti-retinal autoantibodies in VKH syndrome, Behçet's disease and sympathetic ophthalmia. *Ophthalmology*, **92**, 1025–8
35. Manor, R., Livni, E. and Cohen, S. (1979). Cell-mediated immunity to human myelin basic protein in Vogt–Koyanagi–Harada syndrome. *Invest. Ophthalmol. Vis. Sci.*, **18**, 204–6
36. Tagawa, Y. (1978). Lymphocyte mediated cytotoxicity against melanocyte antigen in Vogt–Koyanagi–Harada disease. *Jpn. J. Ophthalmol.*, **22**, 34–39
37. Welch, R., Maumenee, A. and Wahlen, H. (1960). Peripheral posterior segment inflammation, vitreous opacities and oedema of the posterior pole. *Arch. Ophthalmol.*, **64**, 540–9
38. Pruett, R., Brockhurst, R. and Letts, N. (1974). Fluorescein angiography of peripheral uveitis. *Am. J. Ophthalmol.*, **77**, 448–53
39. Ausberger, J., Annesley, W., Sergott, R., Felberg, N., Bowman, J. and Raymond, L. (1981). Familial pars planitis. *Ann. Ophthalmol.*, **13**, 553–7
40. Maumenee, A. (1970). Clinical entities in uveitis. *Trans. Am. Acad. Ophthalmol. Otolaryngol.*, **74**, 473–504
41. Pederson, J., Kenyon, K., Green, R. and Maumenee, E. (1978). Pathology of pars planitis. *Am. J. Ophthalmol.*, **86**, 762–74
42. Kenyon, K., Pederson, J., Green, W. and Maumenee, A. (1975). Fibroglial proliferation in pars planitis. *Trans. Ophthalmol. Soc. U.K.*, **95**, 391–7
43. Wetzig, R., Chan, C., Nussenblatt, R., Palestine, A., Mazur, D. and Mittal, K. (1988). Clinical and immunopathological studies of pars planitis in a family. *Br. J. Ophthalmol.*, **72**, 5–10
44. Roberge, F., Caspi, R., Chan, C., Kuwabara, T. and Nussenblatt, R. (1985). Long term culture of Müller cells from adult rats in the presence of activated lymphocyte/monocyte

97

products. *Curr. Eye Res.*, **4**, 975–82

45. Roberge, F., Caspi, R. and Nussenblatt, R. (1988). Glial retinal cells produce IL-1 activity and have dual effect on autoimmune T-helper lymphocytes. *J. Immunol.*, **140**, 2193–6
46. Mitchell, D., Scadding, J., Heard, B. and Hinson, K. (1977). Sarcoidosis: Histopathological definition and clinical diagnosis. *J. Clin. Pathol.*, **30**, 395–408
47. James, D. (1986). Ocular sarcoidosis. *Ann. N.Y. Acad. Sci.*, **465**, 551–63
48. Gass, J. and Olsen, C. (1973). Sarcoidosis with optic nerve and retinal involvement: a clinicopathological case report. *Trans. Am. Acad. Ophthalmol. Otolaryngol.*, **77**, 739–50
49. Gould, H. and Kaufman, H. (1961). Sarcoid of the fundus. *Arch. Ophthalmol.*, **65**, 453–6
50. Daniele, R., Dauber, J. and Rossman, M. (1980). Immunological abnormalities in sarcoidosis. *Ann. Intern. Med.*, **92**, 406–16
51. Semenzato, G., Agostini, C., Zambello, R. *et al.* (1986). Activated T cells with immunoregulatory functions at different sites of involvement in sarcoidosis. *Ann. N.Y. Acad. Sci.*, **465**, 56–73
52. Chan, C., Wetzig, R., Palestine, A., Kuwabara, T. and Nussenblatt, R. (1987). Immunohistopathology of ocular sarcoidosis. *Arch. Ophthalmol.*, **105**, 1398–402
53. Modlin, R., Hofman, F., Meyer, P., Sharma, O., Taylor, C. and Rea, T. (1983). In situ demonstration of T lymphocyte subsets in granulomatous inflammation. *Clin. Exp. Immunol.*, **51**, 430–8
54. Leung, K. and Ada, G. (1980). Two T cell populations mediate DTH to murine influenza infection. *Scand. J. Immunol.*, **12**, 481–5
55. Hancock, W., Kobzik, L., Colby, A., O'Hara, C., Cooper, A. and Godleski, J. (1986). Detection of lymphokines and lymphokine receptors in pulmonary sarcoidosis. *Am. J. Pathol.*, **123**, 1–8
56. Ohno, S., Kakayama, E., Sugiura, S., Itakura, K., Aoki, K. and Aizawa, M. (1975). Specific histocompatibility antigens associated with Behçet's disease. *Am. J. Ophthalmol.*, **80**, 636
57. Lehner, T., Batchelor, J., Challacombe, S. and Kennedy, L. (1979). An immunogenetic basis for the tissue involvement in Behçet's syndrome. *Immunology*, **37**, 895–900
58. O'Connor, G. (1983). Behçet's disease. In Klein, E. (ed.). Symposium on medical and surgical diseases of the retina and vitreous, pp. 199. (St Louis: Mosby)
59. Eglin, R., Lehner, T. and Subak-Sharpe, J. (1982). Detection of RNA complementary to herpes simplex virus in mononluclear cells from patients with Behçet's syndrome and recurrent oral ulcers. *Lancet*, **2**, 1356–61
60. Bonass, W., Stewart, J., Chamberlain, M. and Halliburton, I. (1986). Molecular studies in Behçet's disease. In Lehner, T. and Barnes, C. (eds.) *Recent Advances in Behçet's Disease*, pp. 37–41. (London: Royal Society of Medicine Services)
61. Mizushima, Y. (1988). Recent research into Behçet's disease in Japan. *Int. J. Tissue Reactions*, **10**, 59–65
62. Miyangana, Y. (1987). *Annual Report of Behçet's Disease Research Committee of Japan*, pp. 181
63. Shimada, K., Yaoita, H. and Shikano, S. (1972). Chemotactic activity in aqueous humour of patients with Behçet's disease. *Jpn. J. Ophthalmol.*, **16**, 84–92
64. Williams, B. and Lehner, T. (1977). Immune complexes in Behçet's syndrome and recurrent oral ulcerations. *Br. Med. J.*, **1**, 1387–9
65. Shimada, K., Kogure, M., Kawashima, T. and Nishioka, K. (1974). Reduction in complement in Behçet's disease and drug allergy. *Med. Biol.*, **52**, 234–9
66. Jorizzo, J., Schmalsteig, F., Solomon, A., Taylor, R. and Cavallo, T. (1986). Studies of circulating immune complexes, neutrophils and effects of oral colchicine or thalidomide in Behçet's disease. In Lehner, T. and Barnes, C. (eds.) *Recent Advances in Behçet's Disease*, pp. 89–96. (London: Royal Society of Medicine Services)
67. Lehner, T. and Barnes, C. (eds.) (1986). *Recent Advances in Behçet's Disease* (London: Royal Society of Medicine Services)
68. Smolin, G. and O'Connor, G. (1986). Immunologic diseases affecting the uveal tract and retina. In *Ocular Immunology*, pp. 312–15 (Boston: Little, Brown and Co.)
69. Yamana, S., Jones, S., Shimamoto, T., Shiota, T., Aoyama, T. and Takasugi, K. (1986). Immunohistological analysis of lymphocytes infiltrating the terminal ileum in a patient with intestinal Behçet's disease. In Lehner, T. and Barnes, C. (eds.) *Recent Advances in Behçet's Disease*, pp. 129–30. (London: Royal Society of Medicine Services)

70. Poulter, L., Lehner, T. and Duke, O. (1985). Immunohistological investigation of recurrent oral ulcers and Behçet's disease. In Lehner, T. and Barnes, C. (eds.) *Recent Advances in Behçet's Disease*, pp. 123–8. (London: Royal Society of Medicine Services)
71. Jongeneel, C., Nedospasov, S., Plaetinck, R., Naquet, P. and Cerottini, J. (1988). Expression of the tumour necrosis factor locus is not necessary for the cytolytic activity of T lymphocytes. *J. Immunol.*, **140**, 1916–22
72. Paliard, X., Malefit, R., Yssel, H., Blanchard, D., Chretien, I., Abrams, J., Vries, J. and Spits, H. (1988). Simultaneous production of IL-2, IL-4 and interferon-γ by activated human CD4+ and CD8+ T-cell clones. *J. Immunol.*, **141**, 849–55

7
Demyelinating Optic Neuropathy

D. A. FRANCIS and W. I. McDONALD

INTRODUCTION

A number of disease processes may give rise to symptoms of optic nerve dysfunction[1], but when these specific causes are excluded there remains a large group of patients in whom the pathology is primarily inflammatory although the aetiology cannot be identified. Within this group the most important cause is demyelinating disease and it is to this particular subgroup that this chapter is addressed. Acute unilateral optic neuritis (ON) affects predominantly the young and middle aged; in 95% of cases the patient is between 16 and 55 years old and onset below 12 years of age is exceptional[2]. The condition shows a female predominance of 2:1 (ref. 3). The incidence of ON is only rarely recorded. Brewis et al.[4] reported an annual incidence rate of 1.4 per 100 000 for ON, compared to 3 per 100 000 for multiple sclerosis (MS), in a northern English town, but both higher and lower frequencies have been reported in other geographical areas that correspond with the local prevalence of MS[5,6].

The first detailed description of acute optic neuritis was given by Nettleship in (1884)[7]. The patient was a 3-year-old boy with total blindness and dilated pupils who recovered completely in 2–3 weeks. Then, as now, the diagnosis was clinical and easily recognized in the typical case. Characteristically, there is a rapid decrease of vision in the affected eye that is generalized but most pronounced centrally. Visual impairment ranges from mild to complete loss, usually reaching its maximum within a few days. Visual symptoms are often preceded by ocular pain, especially on movement of the affected eye, which is thought to be due to distension of the optic nerve sheath. The intensity of the pain has no prognostic value and there is no relationship between the severity of the initial visual loss and the subsequent degree of recovery[8,9]. Recovery is complete in 75–90% of patients[10,11], and usually occurs within 3 months although it may occasionally take longer. Exceptionally, demyelinating optic neuropathy may be recurrent or bilateral and, rarely, the visual loss may be slowly progressive[12]. Subclinical optic neuropathy is frequent, being recognized by asymptomatic pallor of the optic disc, impairment of colour vision, subtle changes in visual fields and contrast sensitivity, insiduous asymptomatic nerve fibre loss[13], or a delayed visual evoked potential (VEP).

The association between idiopathic ON and MS was first noted by Buzzard[14] in 1893 and within a decade ON was recognized as a major cause[15]. It is now well established that up to 75% of patients with MS develop clinical symptoms referable to the optic nerve during the course of their illness and that patients with chronic MS almost invariably show involvement of the anterior visual pathways at postmortem.

PATHOLOGY

The opportunity to examine the optic nerve after an acute attack of isolated ON is rare, and our knowledge of its pathology is derived from the study of patients dying from MS. The predominant pathological feature is demyelination, occurring as plaques, distributed randomly throughout the length of the optic nerve from the scleral canal to the chiasm, with a mean length of about 1 cm[16,17]. Perivascular cuffing with mononuclear cells is commonly seen in regions where there are myelin breakdown products, suggesting recent activity of the disease process. There is evidence that in MS the plaque commences in relation to the venules and expands centrifugally. There is relative preservation of axon continuity, but a variable number of axons usually undergo Wallerian degeneration, resulting in the formation of ophthalmoscopically visible 'slits' or 'grooves' in the retinal nerve fibre layer[13].

Plaques of demyelination tend to persist indefinitely, in spite of good clinical recovery, with limited or no evidence of remyelination, at least in MS. Indirect evidence that remyelination is limited in most adults with ON comes from the persistence of VEP abnormalities in over 90% of patients following clinical resolution[18]. In childhood ON, however, remyelination may be more effective, since the latency of the VEP returned to normal in over half of one series of patients[19]. Chronic demyelinated lesions are characterized by marked astrocytic gliosis in which large numbers of fibrillary astrocytic processes fill the spaces between axons created by myelin loss.

THE RISK OF MULTIPLE SCLEROSIS

The reported frequency with which MS follows ON varies widely (Table 7.1). Several factors probably contribute: patient selection (some studies have been hospital-based while others have relied on military records and yet others on a population base); differences in methods of assessment of patients and in the diagnostic criteria for ON and MS; study design, and duration of follow-up. The much lower frequency in Japanese is consonant with the lower prevalence of MS in Orientals[30]. The overall lower proportion of patients developing MS after ON in most American studies compared to those from Europe initially suggested that there might also be a geographic and/or ethnic effect on risk in caucasoid populations. However, a recent prospective study[24] of 60 patients with ON from New England, USA, has found that overall 58%

Table 7.1 Multiple sclerosis after adult optic neuritis

Study	Observed (%)	Mean period or (range) of follow-up (years)	Predicted (%)
USA			
Taub and Rucker (1954)[20]	32	(10–15)	—
Collis (1965)[21]	36	(7–20)	—
Kurland et al. (1966)[22]	13	(12–18)	—
Cohen et al. (1979)[23]	35	7	—
Rizzo and Lessell (1988)[24]*	58	15	♀74 (by 15 years) ♂34
UK			
Lynn (1959)[25]	50	(0.3–29)	—
McAlpine (1964)[26]†	85	(6–29)	—
Bradley and Whitty (1968)[27]	51	10	—
Hutchinson (1976)[8]	51	8	78 (by 15 years)
Perkins and Rose (1979)[3]	58	(0.2–5.5)	—
Compston et al. (1978)[28]	40	4	60 (by 8 years)
Francis et al. (1987)[29]‡	57	11.6	75 (by 15 years)

*Review of Cohen et al. (1979) patients
†Review of Lynn's data
‡Review of Compston et al. (1978) patients

will have developed MS 15 years after their attack of ON; this figure is comparable to the most recently observed rate in the UK of 57% after almost 12 years[29]. When allowance for variations in length of follow-up were computed the risk approached 75%.

A number of factors associated with an increased risk of developing MS after ON have been identified within individual patient groups.

Age and sex

Rizzo and Lessell found a much higher risk for subsequent development of MS in females than in males (69% vs 33%)[24]. They also found that onset of ON between the ages of 21 and 40 years had a modest effect on increasing the risk of developing MS that was more pronounced in females ($p < 0.03$). A greater relative risk of progression to MS in females has been reported by several investigators (Table 7.2), although in each study female patients with ON outnumbered males. Taub and Rucker also found that the risk was marginally increased in those over the age of 20 years compared to younger patients, but with no sex difference[20].

Optic neuritis is uncommon in childhood but when it occurs is more often bilateral. The future risk of developing MS in such cases appears to be low, between 5 and 15%[19,32]. The prognosis should be more guarded in children with unilateral involvement. Five patients in Kennedy and Carter's series with unilateral childhood ON later developed MS[33] and in a more recent series 3

Table 7.2 Optic neuritis progression to multiple sclerosis according to sex

Study	Percentage developing MS		Relative risk for females
	Female	Male	
Cohen *et al.* (1979)[23]	45(19/42)	11(2/18)	4.1
Kinnunen (1983)[6]	20(40/201)	9.5(9/95)	2.1
Hely *et al.* (1986)[31]	38(23/59)	13(3/23)	2.8
Rizzo and Lessell (1988)[24]*	69(29/42)	33(6/18)	3.4

*Review of Cohen *et al.* (1979) patients

out of 10 patients with uniocular disease subsequently developed neurological symptoms outside the visual pathway[19].

Recurrence

Recurrence represents a further episode of neurological disturbance and occurs in at least one-fifth of patients depending on the length of follow-up. The data of Compston *et al.*[28] and Cohen *et al.*[23] suggested that the risk of developing lesions elsewhere in the central nervous system was increased by

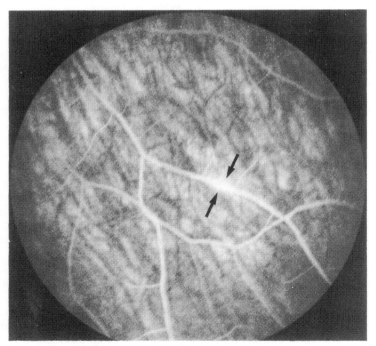

Figure 7.1 Fluorescein angiogram showing focal leakage of fluorescein dye (arrows) from a retinal vessel of a patient with optic neuritis

recurrence of ON in the same or the other eye, but such a high proportion of patients ultimately developed MS in these studies that later follow-up failed to confirm the effect[24,29] in keeping with other reports[8,31].

Retinal perivascular sheathing

As described below, ophthalmoscopically visible peripheral perivenular sheathing or focal fluorescein leakage (Figure 7.1) is visible in about a quarter of patients at presentation and significantly increases the risk of later development of MS ($p < 0.02$; relative risk, R.R. $= 14.4$)[34].

Oligoclonal IgG bands (OB) in the cerebrospinal fluid (CSF)

There have been several reports that the presence of oligoclonal IgG bands on immunoelectrophoresis of the CSF of patients indicates an increased risk for the subsequent development of MS (R.R. $= 3.2$[35]) after episodes of isolated clinical syndromes including ON[35,36]. The relevance of this will be discussed later.

Histocompatibility antigen association

The predictive value of particular HLA antigens is at present unclear and is also discussed further below.

Asymptomatic dissemination

Sanders *et al.*, using various tests, found objective abnormalities in the CNS outside of the visual pathway in 11 (37%) of 30 patients presenting with isolated ON[37]. The abnormalities included increased latency of auditory and somatosensory EPs, abnormal blink reflexes and electronystagmography, and other lesions demonstrated on CT scanning. A much higher frequency (60–70%) has been found by magnetic resonance (MRI) scanning (Figure 7.2). The presence of such lesions at presentation greatly increases the risk of development of MS within 1 year ($p < 0.005$; RR $= 6.8$[38]).

Serial MRI has revealed a high frequency of asymptomatic new lesions in patients either with isolated clinical syndromes such as ON, or with MS. Current figures for the risk of development of MS in relation to the particular clinical or investigative features already mentioned are thus likely to be an underestimate.

IMMUNOLOGICAL ABNORMALITIES

Several lines of evidence now indicate that demyelination in patients with ON (and MS) is immunologically mediated (reviewed in ref. 39). However, it is still not clear which of the recognized immunological disturbances are primary events and important in the subsequent development of the lesions.

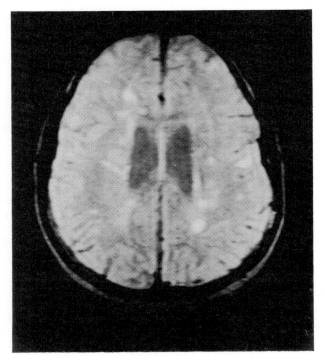

Figure 7.2 SE$_{2000/60}$ axial magnetic resonance image showing multiple periventricular and focal cerebral white matter lesions in a patient with isolated acute unilateral optic neuritis

Genetic susceptibility

The familial aggregation of patients with MS has been known since the latter part of the last century[40] and an increased incidence of monosymptomatic demyelination, particularly ON, in multiple-case MS families has recently been emphasized[41]. Sophisticated pedigree analysis has established the role of a genetic factor in the aetiology of MS and most work over the last two decades has centred on the close association between the disease and certain MHC-region (HLA) tissue markers. It is likely, however, that more than one gene — not necessarily on the same chromosome — is involved.

The major histocompatibility complex (MHC)

The human major histocompatibility complex (MHC), or HLA region, is located on the short arm of chromosome 6 and is divided into three classes of genes; Class I, histocompatibility antigens (HLA-A, HLA-B and HLA-C); Class II, immune response genes (HLA-DP, HLA-DQ and HLA-DR); and Class III, complement components (C4, C2 and Bf)[42]. The usual explanation for HLA-associated disease invokes close linkage to a putative disease

106

susceptibility gene, or genes, situated within or near the HLA loci on the sixth chromosome. The known biological functions of the HLA system may also play in important role. For example, it is known that the presence of individual HLA-gene products or linked haplotypes influences patterns of immune responsiveness in certain individuals to both foreign and self-antigen[43]. Under appropriate environmental conditions these might lower the threshold for establishing an immunological process that results in the later development of clinical disease.

Following the earliest HLA-MS studies, it is now clear that patients from Northern caucasian populations show strongest association with the Class II antigen, HLA-DR2 (present in 50–55% of patients). The initial weak associations with HLA-A3 and HLA-B7 occurred because of their strong biological linkage with HLA-DR2[44]. Although this antigen has shown closest correlation with MS in most European studies to date[44], no significant association was noted between HLA-DR2 and patients from both the Grampian region of Scotland[45] and the Orkney Islands[46]. HLA-DQw1, on the other hand, when sought in the former population was significantly increased[45], raising the possibility that, in certain populations, other HLA markers may lie in close linkage with one of the putative MS susceptibility genes. This suggestion is supported by similar HLA Class II differences reported in several ethnic groups around the world[47,48].

A similar distribution of HLA antigens has been found in patients with ON. Sandberg-Wollheim et al. reported associations with HLA-A3, HLA-B7 and HLA-Ld 7a (equivalent to Dw2 and linked to DR2) that were as strong as those noted in patients with MS[49]. They concluded that the two conditions represented different aspects of the same disease. In common with most other studies[28,50] we have found an intermediate frequency of HLA-DR2 in our patients with ON in the South-East of England that remains significantly different from normal individuals[29]. In the study by Compston et al., 146 patients who had presented with isolated ON up to 23 years before were investigated retrospectively[28]. Forty per cent had developed MS at review (mean follow-up 47 months) and a high proportion of these cases was positive for 'BT 101', a locally designated Class II antigen broadly equivalent to DR2 and DQw1. The presence of this antigen was associated with an increased risk (R.R. = 3.95) of developing MS. Sixty per cent of the original ON group developed MS after longer follow-up (mean 11.6 years)[29], but in this more recent review neither HLA-DR2 nor HLA-DQw1 were significant predictive risk factors. This discrepancy may be partly explained both by the use of newer reagents and techniques in the second study, allowing more accurate typing, and by the failure to incorporate all patients from the original survey. In the only prospective study to date to report the influence of HLA type on the risk of developing MS in individuals with ON (mean follow-up 57 months) HLA-DR2 positivity did appear to increase the risk (R.R. = 2.7)[31]. The established association of HLA-DR2 with ON, considering the strong connection between this marker and MS, points to a common predisposing genetic factor. In our study, when the period of observation was extended, several HLA-DR2 negative individuals also developed MS[29]. It is therefore important to remember that the absence of this, or any other associated HLA antigen, does not preclude the subsequent development of disseminated disease.

Other HLA region gene products have been studied in relation to MS and ON. Fielder *et al.* investigated the frequencies of Factor B (Bf) alleles in three groups of British patients with isolated ON, suspected MS and clinically definite MS (CDMS), respectively[51]. The frequency of HLA-DR2 was similar in all three groups and in each case significantly higher than in the control population, confirming previous observations. The allele Bf*F, however, was significantly under-represented in the group of patients with CDMS when compared to the other two groups. Their explanation of these findings was that HLA-DR2, as a marker of susceptibility to demyelination in general, would occur equally in all three groups, whereas variations in the distribution of alleles of the Bf system might confer differences in the rate of progression to MS, possibly through influences on the complement system (see later). The influence of Bf alleles on either the development or progression of MS has not been confirmed in subsequent groups of patients studied retrospectively by the same laboratory[29,45] or by other investigators[52].

The close relationship between ON and MS is undisputed, but the different HLA frequencies noted between the two groups does suggest that causative immunological factors may be influenced to a varying degree, resulting in some, but not all, patients with ON progressing to MS.

Immunoglobulin abnormalities

Qualitative and quantitative changes in immunoglobulins, particularly of the IgG class, are well documented in the cerebrospinal fluid (CSF) of patients with MS[53]; although their specificity and target antigen(s) are unknown. CSF abnormalities have also been described in patients with ON in the form of discrete oligoclonal IgG bands on immunoelectrophoresis[36] or less frequently by evidence of increased intrathecal IgG synthesis[53]. These changes are comparable to those in established MS. Moulin *et al.*[35] found that 24% of 83 patients with isolated demyelinating lesions and abnormal CSF protein electrophoresis (including 11 cases with ON) developed definite MS during follow-up, compared to 9 out of 100 patients who did not have an oligoclonal pattern on CSF electrophoresis (including 21 cases with ON). Other studies correlating clinical dissemination with the presence of CSF oligoclonal bands in patients with ON have supported this finding[54,55], whereas Sandberg-Wollheim, in a prospective study, concluded that there was no predictive value because a substantial proportion of her patients with ON and no oligoclonal bands in the CSF also developed MS[36].

The antigenic specificity of IgG present in CSF from patients with demyelinating lesions has not been elucidated to date but is generally thought to reflect the consequences of chronic CNS inflammation resulting in the activation of restricted B-cell subpopulations released from normal suppressor mechanisms. An alternative explanation centres around the possibility of a viral aetiology. Indirect correlations between the presence of oligoclonal bands and antibodies to measles[53], mumps, rubella and herpes simplex[56] have been claimed, but it is accepted that even in combination these viral antibodies account for only a small fraction of the total CSF IgG present in patients with demyelinating disease.

Sandberg-Wollheim et al., reporting on 54 patients with ON, described a correlation between HLA-A3 and oligoclonal bands in CSF, but not between HLA-B7 or Dw2[49]. Conversely, Stendahl-Brodin et al. (1978) found that the frequency of HLA-Dw2 in patients with ON and oligoclonal bands in CSF was of a magnitude similar to that seen in MS[50]. It seems probable that there is an association between the presence of oligoclonal IgG and MS-associated HLA antigens but that it is not complete, for reasons that are poorly understood.

Gm allotypes

Human immunoglobulin (Ig) consists of two heavy and two light chains. Variations in heavy-chain structure are genetically controlled and those for the IgG class are coded by Gm allotypes, a system of limited polymorphism, located on chromosome 14. Herein may lie one of the other genetic factors influencing susceptibility to MS. Several reports indicate that variations in Gm allotypic expression appear to confer differences in immunological function that result in susceptibility to certain diseases[57,58]. The observed abnormalities of IgG production within the CNS of patients with demyelinating disease have therefore stimulated interest in the distribution of Gm alleles. Two independent studies have suggested that the Gm phenotype (1, 17; 21) carries an increased risk for the development of MS in caucasians (R.R. = 3.6)[59,60]. A different but equally strong association was found in a large population of patients with MS from north-east Scotland, an area of high prevalence of the disease[61]. In this population there was a significant positive association between the Gm phenotype Gm (3; 5), the presence of HLA-DQw1 and disease occurrence ($p < 0.01$; R.R. = 3.3). Gm 3; 5 was also significantly increased among MS patients from the Hautes-Pyrenees in France (R.R. = 2.4)[62]. This particular Gm haplotype has been found with increased frequency in other autoimmune diseases[63] and evidence is accumulating from other centres that genes for both the MHC and Gm systems may interact to influence susceptibility to this group of diseases[64].

The distribution of Gm allotypes in ON is poorly documented. In a recent Swedish study[65], the CSF and serum from 64 patients with MS and 47 patients with isolated ON were analysed for Gm alleles. While significantly increased frequencies of Gm 1; 21 and Gm 1, 2; 21 were found in the MS patient group (R.R. = 2.1), the distribution among patients with ON did not differ from normal individuals.

The conflicting reports on Gm allotype distribution in MS suggest that Gm influences in this condition are primarily immune-mediated rather than secondary to close proximity to disease-susceptibility gene markers. The lack of any association between MS and alleles of the PI system, which is in strong linkage disequilibrium with Gm loci on chromosome 14, supports this view[66].

Genetic influences on monosymptomatic ON require further investigation but it seems feasible that interactive and/or additive effects of two, or more, immunogenetic systems that govern different populations of lymphocytes, (i.e. Gm allotypes, B cells; HLA Class II antigens, T cells) may augment susceptibility to a multifactorial disease such as MS.

Complement abnormalities

In addition to variations in the distribution of MHC-linked complement alleles, abnormalities in serum and CSF complement pathway profiles have been reported in MS and ON. Most studies have examined the early components of the complement cascade. Elevated C3 CSF levels with normal C4 values were reported by Yam et al.[67], raising the possibility of release from inflammatory cells, e.g. macrophages, as part of a cell-activation process. However, Compston[68] has pointed out that many of the early components of the complement cascade are resynthesized locally within the central nervous system, making reported changes in CSF concentration difficult to interpret. To overcome this problem, he measured the CSF concentration of C9, the terminal component of complement and an integral part of the membrane attack complex, which is predominantly synthesized in the liver. He argued that changes in the CSF concentration of this component were more likely to indicate evidence of complement activation and deposition at sites of CNS damage. As part of a larger study of CSF and plasma C9 concentration in patients with MS[69], these investigators included seven patients with monosymptomatic ON (although three had evidence of previous neurological involvement). They found, as in patients with disseminated disease, an overall reduction in the CSF C9 index (CSF/plasma ratio) that supported their hypothesis of IgG-mediated activation of the classical complement pathway in the pathogenesis of demyelination. Two types of demyelinating lesion were postulated[68]: the first in which complement-activating immune complexes have formed in sufficient concentration to damage myelin irreversibly, thereby causing persistent morphological changes; and a second, milder, lesion in which increased membrane permeability would alter thresholds of axonal conduction already compromised by partial demyelination. This second lesion could be associated with the common transient clinical abnormalities and the potential for full recovery of function.

These are attractive hypotheses, but one must remember that, although such changes may represent specific complement activation initiated by the binding of antibodies directed against certain CNS constituents, they may represent non-specific complement activation occurring as a result of immunological damage.

Abnormalities in lymphocyte subpopulations

T-cell subpopulations play an integral role with MHC molecules in cellular immunity and can be recognized and enumerated by means of monoclonal antibodies to the cell surface antigens, most commonly OKT4/CD4 and OKT8/CD8. Cell-mediated lesions are initiated by antigen-specific T cells of the helper/inducer phenotype (OKT4+). Class II antigens (DR, DQ) of the MHC are important in these reactions as the T cell must recognize antigen presented to it in combination with the host's Class II products in order for it to be activated and thereby activate other cells, e.g. macrophages. Other

T-cell functions are mediated by antigen-specific OKT8+ T cells that cause cytotoxic reactions only if the target cell bears Class I (HLA A, B, Cw) MHC antigens of the same specificity. Finally the ability to develop specific suppressor T-cell responses may be under Class II gene control[70].

The earliest evidence concerning the influence of lymphocyte subpopulations in MS suggested a reduction in circulating cytotoxic/suppressor T lymphocytes in patients with either active or progressive disease[71,72]. The observations were based on single measurements but were confirmed by serial studies in individual patients[73]. However, others have failed to show consistent changes in active disease and similar reductions in circulating OKT8+ cells have been noted in normal individuals and patients with the quiescent form of MS[74,75].

The relative proportions of T and B lymphocytes were normal in the few studies on peripheral blood from patients with ON; whereas "activated" T cells and total B-cell counts appear to be reduced in CSF, although this did not correlate with disease activity[76,77]. Compston, enumerating circulating peripheral blood lymphocytes in 22 patients with ON within a month of onset of visual symptoms (7 patients had concomitant or previous neurological signs) found that overall the number of OKT8+ cells was reduced[73]. Serial observations in a proportion of these patients showed a return of the OKT4/8 ratio to normal, again independently of any symptomatic recovery, in the majority of patients with isolated ON, but fluctuating levels in those associated with other neurological signs consistent with MS.

The explanation for the observed decrease in suppressor/cytotoxic cells in the blood of patients with MS, when observed, and the transient reduction noted in ON is not clear. Taken overall, there is a poor correlation between the circulating population of OKT8+ cells and suppressor function in patients with MS[78] and this may be because measuring peripheral blood lymphocytes gives only an indirect impression of regulatory mechanisms occurring within the CNS. Migration of OKT8+ cells into the CNS is one suggested cause, although not all studies of CSF cell subpopulations support this view[79] and not all groups have found a predominance of OKT8+ cells in MS lesions[80]. One postulated alternative suggests that defective suppressor function might reflect persistent alteration in the properties of OKT8+ cells rather than changes in the actual number of cells involved[81]. Other parameters of cellular function, for example the noted reduction in natural killer (NK) cell activity and interferon production in MS[82], provide evidence for a generalized abnormality in immunoregulatory activity rather than a specific role for these cells in the absence of an identifiable CNS antigen. As new, and even more specific, generations of monoclonal antibodies are developed, these discrepancies may be resolved.

PATHOGENESIS

Owing to its benign outcome in the majority of patients, little direct information is available about the pathogenesis of optic neuritis, although its close association with MS allows some reasonable conjectures. There are

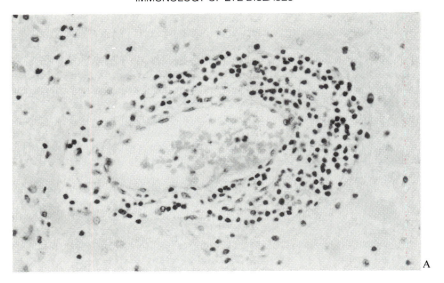

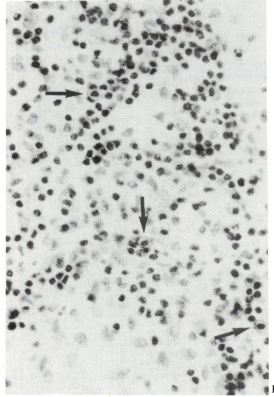

unquestionable alterations in the immune system of patients with active demyelination and the presence of enhancing plaques demonstrated by contrast-enhanced computer tomography and MRI has been widely accepted as evidence of alterations of the blood–brain barrier (BBB) and representative of disease activity[17,83–85]. The close association of enhancement with gadolinium–DTPA and histological evidence of active inflammation in the immune-mediated experimental disease chronic relapsing experimental allergic encephalomyelitis (EAE), which has important morphological similarities to the lesion of MS and ON, suggest that these changes may be causally related to the development of the lesion (Hawkins *et al.* unpublished).

The early lesion

Early plaques of demyelination are characterized by the presence of intracellular and extracellular myelin debris and an overall increase in cellularity. These lesions are characteristically orientated around venules, the walls of which are infiltrated by mononuclear cells forming perivascular cuffs that include lymphocytes and plasma cells[86,87] (Figure 7.3). Prineas and his colleagues[88] have suggested that this results from a direct cellular attack on the myelin sheath rather than from a primary degeneration of the myelin-forming oligodendrocyte. They have described myelin breakdown occurring in close relationship to phagocytic cells and the incorporation of myelin lamellae into macrophage processes though this observation awaits confirmation. The oligodendrocyte is, however, affected at some stage, since the overall number of such cells appears to be reduced within the lesion[89].

Retinal venous sheathing has long been associated with MS[90] and is probably the visible correlation of perivascular cuffing in acute lesions, representing the earliest manifestation of the pathological process, which occurs in the white matter of the optic nerve in ON or elsewhere in the CNS in MS. Recently, we have obtained evidence for the occurrence of inflammatory changes in the retina of 14 out of 50 consecutive patients presenting with acute idiopathic optic neuritis[34]. Fifty-seven per cent of the patients with sheathing and/or uveitis have subsequently developed clinical evidence of MS over a mean follow-up period of 3.5 years, compared to 14% of patients with no retinal vascular abnormalities. These macroscopic appearances in a region free of myelin and oligodendrocytes support Prineas' suggestion that the vascular changes in MS are primary, and not secondary to myelin breakdown.

At a functional level, the recent use of monoclonal antibodies has shown that, in addition to a preponderance of CD4+ T-helper cells within perivascular cuffs[91], there are infiltrations of activated T lymphocytes in the 'normal-appearing' white matter adjacent to the edge of active plaques[92].

◀ **Figure 7.3** (A) Photomicrograph of a small vein within a plaque. The vessel is cuffed by an irregular grouping of small cells most of which are lymphocytes. The surrounding brain tissue shows marked glial proliferation. (H & E stain, ×300). (B) Immunocytochemical stain for T lymphocytes, using MT1 antibody, shows faint reaction in some perivascular cells (arrows) (×480)

Fontana et al.[93] have shown that astrocytes in culture are capable of expressing MHC Class II antigens and Traugott[94] has demonstrated both Class II-positive astrocytes and endothelial cells in active MS lesions. The presence of Class II MHC antigens on CNS vascular endothelium might facilitate the passage of activated T cells into cerebral white matter that has been noted in studies on EAE in mice[95] and more recently in patients with progressive MS[96]. The preferential transfer of Class II MHC-restricted helper T cells into this normally immuno-privileged site would expose myelin to potential mechanisms of breakdown.

Tissue damage, in EAE, can be initiated by a T-cell response to various myelin antigens, most notably myelin basic protein (MBP)[97]; although neither the presence of these encephalitogenic T cells nor their reactivity correlates well with the clinical course of the disease model[98] invoking other immunological mechanisms. Furthermore, T-cell clones of various phenotypes (cytotoxic, helper and suppressor) from the blood and CSF of patients with MS have failed to show significant reactivity against MBP and other major myelin proteins[99], suggesting that these responses are not critical in the pathogenesis of MS in man. Recent evidence correlates disease activity in EAE more closely with BBB dysfunction[100], re-emphasizing the importance of the CNS vascular endothelium, which in turn relies on the normal functioning of supporting astrocytes for its integrity[101]. Damage to either cell type as a result of Class II expression would increase BBB permeability to inflammatory cells. The precise relationship between these initial inflammatory events and subsequent demyelination in ON, or MS, remains unclear. Macrophages appear to be the final vectors of myelin destruction, as reaffirmed by Prineas in electron-microscopic studies, possibly by receptor-mediated endocytosis[89]. Dense infiltrations of Class II positive macrophages have been found at the centre of actively demyelinating plaques[94] that may have been triggered by activated CD4+ T lymphocytes.

Overall, it seems likely that Class II MHC antigen expression has a prime role in the local presentation of antigen to activated T-cell lines preferentially sequestered within the CNS and directed against a heterogeneous array of CNS constituents. Class II antigen modulation of both vascular endothelium and supporting astrocytes represents an early event in pathogenesis of demyelination, resulting in alterations in the BBB. The mechanisms that promote this aberrant expression in the first place remain to be elucidated.

TREATMENT

The strong evidence that many cases of ON are mediated immunologically provides a rationale for immunosuppressant therapy. However, the need for treatment in acute optic neuritis is controversial because of the excellent prognosis for vision in most patients. This has resulted in only a limited number of prospective studies with comparable patient groups.

Rawson et al.[102] and Rawson and Liversedge[103] carried out a double-blind trial of treatment with ACTH in acute ON. A faster recovery was noted in the treated group than in the control patients after 30 days, but 2 years after the

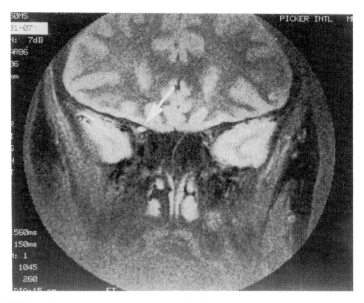

Figure 7.4 Magnetic resonance scan: coronal orbital image ($IR_{1560/150/40}$) in a patient with right optic neuritis. There is increased signal within the right optic nerve (arrowed)

onset no significant differences in visual acuity were noted between treated and untreated patients. Similar prospective studies by Bowden et al.[104] and by Gould et al.[9] (in the latter, triamcinolone was administered by retrobulbar injection) again showed a faster recovery but no significant difference in final acuity after up to 24 months of follow-up. It seems likely that, although the acute phase of the disease may be shortened, the final outcome of ON is not influenced by ACTH or steroid treatment alone in most patients, though it may be pointed out that the natural recovery rate is so high that much larger studies than those so far conducted would be needed to demonstrate a real if infrequent beneficial effect. Schmidt recommends steroid therapy, if ophthalmological examination reveals oedema of the optic nerve head, in order to prevent hypothetical secondary ischaemic damage to nerve fibres compressed within the narrowed confines of the lamina cribosa-scleral The finding of a significant association between failure to recover and the presence of MRI-detected lesions in the optic canal[17] (Figure 7.4) raises the question of whether patients with such lesions might benefit from steroid treatment. A prospective controlled study is clearly needed. In the light of existing evidence, it is appropriate to treat patients with bilateral involvement or those in whom vision is already poor in the unaffected eye in order to achieve a more rapid improvement in visual acuity of the affected eye.

The use of other immunosuppressant agents in demyelinating disease has proved disappointing. Current interest has centred around two therapeutic alternatives. The interferons have been used to stimulate immune responses in MS. The theoretical risk that treatment with interferon-γ (which *increases*

Class II MHC antigen expression) might induce exacerbations in patients with MS, particularly after viral infections (which themselves induce endogenous interferon-γ production), was realized in one recent therapeutic study[106]; whereas interferon-β (which *reduces* Class II expression) has shown some promise in early trials[107]. Secondly, whereas whole or fragmentary MBP induces EAE in animals, Copolymer 1 — a synthetic polypeptide sequence of MBP that is non-toxic and non-encephalitogenic — is capable of suppressing the disease by desensitization. Although MBP does not appear to influence the course of MS in man, Copolymer 1 has been used with some success in both relapsing–remitting and chronic progressive forms of the disease[108] and the results of an extended trial are soon to be published.

References

1. Heron, J. R. (1985). Diagnosis of optic neuropathy. In Hess, R. F. and Plant, G. J. (eds.). *Optic Neuritis*, pp. 51–71. (Cambridge: Cambridge University Press)
2. Russell, R. W. S. (1983). Symptomatology of optic neuritis. *Bull. Soc. Belge Ophtal.*, **208—I**, 127–30
3. Perkins, G. D. and Rose, F. C. (eds.) (1979). *Optic Neuritis and its Differential Diagnosis*, pp. 292. (Oxford: Oxford University Press)
4. Brewis, M., Poskanzer, D. C., Rolland, C. and Miller, H. (1965). Neurological disease in an English city. *Acta Neurol. Scand.*, **42**, suppl. 24, 1–89
5. Poskanzer, D. C., Prenney, L. B., Sheridan, J. L. and Yon Kondy, J. (1980). Multiple sclerosis in the Orkney and Shetland Islands. (1) Epidemiology, clinical factors, and methodology. *J. Epidemiol. Commun. Health*, **34**, 229–39
6. Kinnunen, E. (1983). The incidence of optic neuritis and its prognosis for multiple sclerosis. *Acta Neurol. Scand.*, **68**, 371–7
7. Nettleship, E. (1884). On cases of retro ocular neuritis. *Trans. Ophthalmol. Soc. U.K.*, **4**, 186–226
8. Hutchinson, W. M. (1976). Acute optic neuritis and the prognosis for multiple sclerosis. *J. Neurol. Neurosurg. Psychiatry*, **39**, 283–9
9. Gould, E. S., Bird, A. C., Leaver, P. K. and McDonald, W. I. (1977). Treatment of optic neuritis by retrobulbar injection of triamcinolone. *Br. Med. J.*, **1**, 1495–7
10. Bradley, W. G. and Whitty, C. W. M. (1967). Acute optic neuritis: its clinical features and their relation to prognosis for recovery of vision. *J. Neurol. Neurosurg. Psychiatry*, **30**, 531–8
11. Earl, C. J. and Martin, B. (1967). Prognosis in optic neuritis related to age. *Lancet*, **1**, 74–6
12. Ormerod, I. E. C. and McDonald, W. I. (1984). Multiple sclerosis presenting with progressive visual failure. *J. Neurol. Neurosurg. Psychiatry*, **47**, 943–6
13. Frisén, L. and Hoyt, W. F. (1974). Insidious atrophy of retinal nerve fibres in multiple sclerosis. *Arch. Ophthalmol.*, **92**, 91–7
14. Buzzard, T. (1893). Atrophy of the optic nerve as a symptom of chronic disease of the central nervous system. *Br. Med. J.*, **2**, 779–84
15. Gunn, R. M. (1904). Retro ocular neuritis. *Lancet*, **2**, 412.
16. McDonald, W. I. (1977). Pathophysiology of conduction in central nerve fibres. In Desmedt, J. E. (ed.) *Visual Evoked Potentials in Man*, pp. 427–37. (Oxford: Clarendon Press)
17. Miller, D. H., Rudge, P., Johnson, G., Kendall, B. E., MacManus, D. G., Moseley, I. F., Barnes, D. and McDonald, W. I. (1988). Serial gadolinium enhanced magnetic resonance imaging in multipe sclerosis. *Brain*, **111**, 927–39
18. Halliday, A. M. (ed.) (1982). *Evoked Potentials in Clinical Testing*, pp. 211 (Edinburgh: Churchill Livingstone)
19. Kriss, A., Francis, D. A., Cuendet, F., Halliday, A. M., Taylor, D. S. I., Wilson, J., Keast-Butler, J., Batchelor, J. R. and McDonald, W. I. (1988). Recovery after optic neuritis in childhood. *J. Neurol. Neurosurg. Psychiatry*, **51**, 1253–8

20. Taub, R. G. and Rucker, C. W. (1954). The relationship of retrobulbar neuritis to multiple sclerosis. *Am. J. Ophthalmol.*, **37**, 494–7
21. Collis, W. J. (1965). Acute unilateral retrobulbar neuritis. *Arch. Neurol.*, **13**, 409–12
22. Kurland, L. T., Beebe, G. W., Kurtzke, J. F., Nagler, B., Auth, T. L., Lessell, S. and Nefziger, M. D. (1966). Studies on the natural history of multiple sclerosis. 2. The progression of optic neuritis to multiple sclerosis. *Acta Neurol. Scand.*, **42**, Suppl. 19, 157–76
23. Cohen, M. M., Lessell, S. and Wolf, P. A. (1979). A prospective study of the risk of developing multiple sclerosis in uncomplicated optic neuritis. *Neurology (Minneap.)*, **29**, 208–13
24. Rizzo, J. F. and Lessell, S. (1988). Risk of developing multiple sclerosis after uncomplicated optic neuritis: a long term prospective study. *Neurology*, **38**, 185–90
25. Lynn, B. H. (1959). Retrobulbar neuritis. *Trans. Ophthal. Soc. U.K.*, **79**, 701–16
26. McAlpine, D. (1964). The benign form of multiple sclerosis: results of a long-term study. *Br. Med. J.*, **2**, 1029–32
27. Bradley, W. G. and Whitty, C. W. M. (1968). Acute optic neuritis: prognosis for development of multiple sclerosis. *J. Neurol. Neurosurg. Psychiatry*, **31**, 10–18
28. Compston, D. A. S., Batchelor, J. R., Earl, C. J. and McDonald, W. I. (1978). Factors influencing the risk of multiple sclerosis developing in patients with optic neuritis. *Brain*, **101**, 495–511
29. Francis, D. A., Compston, D. A. S., Batchelor, J. R. and McDonald, W. I. (1987). A reassessment of the risk of multiple sclerosis developing in patients with optic neuritis after extended follow-up. *J. Neurol. Neurosurg. Psychiatry*, **50**, 758–65
30. Isayama, Y., Takahashi, T., Shimoyoma, T. and Yamadori, A. (1982). Acute optic neuritis and multiple sclerosis. *Neurology (N.Y.)*, **32**, 73–6
31. Hely, M. A., McManis, P. G., Doran, T. J., Walsh, J. C. and McLeod, J. G. (1986). Acute optic neuritis: a prospective study of risk factors for multiple sclerosis. *J. Neurol. Neurosurg. Psychiatry*, **49**, 1125–30
32. Parkin, P. J., Hierons, R. and McDonald, W. I. (1984). Bilateral optic neuritis: a long term follow-up. *Brain*, **107**, 951–64
33. Kennedy, C. and Carter, S. (1961). Relation of optic neuritis to multiple sclerosis in children. *Paediatrics*, **28**, 377–87
34. Lightman, S., McDonald, W. I., Bird, A. C., Francis, D. A., Hoskins, A., Batchelor, J. R. and Halliday, A. M. (1987). Retinal venous sheathing in optic neuritis: its significance for the pathogenesis of multiple sclerosis. *Brain*, **110**, 405–14
35. Moulin, D., Paty, D. W. and Ebers, G. C. (1983). The predictive value of cerebrospinal fluid electrophoresis in 'possible' multiple sclerosis. *Brain*, **106**, 809–16
36. Sandberg-Wollheim, M. (1975). Optic neuritis: studies on the cerebrospinal fluid in relation to clinical course in 61 patients. *Acta Neurol. Scand.*, **52** 167–78
37. Sanders, E., Reulen, J. P. H. and Hogenhuis, L. A. H. (1984). Central nervous system involvement in optic neuritis. *J. Neurol. Neurosurg. Psychiatry*, **47**, 241–9
38. Miller, D. H., Ormerod, I. E. C., McDonald, W. I., MacManus, D. G., Kendall, B. E., Kingsley, D. P. E. and Moseley, I. F. (1988). The early risk of multiple sclerosis after optic neuritis. *J. Neurol. Neurosurg. Psychiatry*, **51**, 1569–71
39. McDonald, W. I. (1983). Doyne lecture: the significance of optic neuritis. *Trans. Ophthalmol. Soc. U.K.*, **103**, 230–46
40. Gowers, W. R. (ed.) (1888). *A Manual of Diseases of the Nervous System*, Vol. 2, p. 507. (London: J. and A. Churchill)
41. Ebers, G. C., Cousin, H. K., Feasby, T. E. and Paty, D. W. (1981). Optic neuritis in familial MS. *Neurology*, **31**, 1138–42
42. Barnstable, C. J., Jones, E. A. and Crumpton, M. J. (1978). Isolation, structure and genetics of HLA-A, B, C, and DRw(Ia) antigens. *Br. Med. Bull.*, **34**, 241–6
43. Bennacerraf, B. (1981). Role of MHC gene products in immune regulation. *Science*, **212**, 1229–38
44. Batchelor, J. R. (1985). Immunological and genetic aspects of multiple sclerosis. In Matthews, W. B., Acheson, E. D., Batchelor, J. R. and Weller, R. O. (eds.) *McAlpines Multiple Sclerosis*, pp. 281–300 (London: Churchill Livingstone)
45. Francis, D. A., Batchelor, J. R., McDonald, W. I., Hing, S. N., Dodi, I. A., Fielder, A. H.

L., Hern, J. E. C. and Downie, A. W. (1987). Multiple sclerosis in north-east Scotland. An association with HLA-DQw1. *Brain*, **110**, 181–96

46. Poskanzer, D. C., Terasaki, P. I., Prenney, L. B., Sheridan, J. L. and Park, M. S. (1980). Multiple sclerosis in the Orkney and Shetland Islands. III. Histocompatibility determinants. *J. Epidemiol. Commun. Health.*, **34**, 253–7

47. Kurdi, A., Ayesh, I., Abdallat, A., Maayta, U., McDonald, W. I., Compston, D. A. S. and Batchelor, J. R. (1977). Different B lymphocyte alloantigens associated with multiple sclerosis in Arabs and North Europeans. *Lancet*, **1**, 1123–5

48. Naito, S., Takeshi, T. and Kuroiwa, Y. (1982). HLA studies of multiple sclerosis in Japan. In Kuroiwa, Y. and Kurland, L. T. (eds.) *Multiple Sclerosis. East and West*, pp. 215–22 (Basel and London: Karger)

49. Sandberg-Wollheim, M., Platz, P., Ryder, L., Nielsen, L. and Thompsen, M. (1975). HL-A histocompatibility antigens in optic neuritis. *Acta. Neurol. Scand.*, **52**, 161–6

50. Stendahl-Brodin, L., Link, H., Moller, E. and Norrby, E. (1978). Optic neuritis and distribution of genetic markers of the HLA system. *Acta Neurol. Scand.*, **53**, 418–31

51. Fielder, A. H. L., Batchelor, J. R., Vakarelis, B. N., Compston, D. A. S. and McDonald, W. I. (1981). Optic neuritis and multiple sclerosis: do Factor B alleles influence progression of disease? *Lancet*, **2**, 1246–8

52. Bertrams, J., Grosse-Wilde, H. and Kuwert, E. (1981). Normal distribution of Factor B (Bf) allotypes in multiple sclerosis. *J. Neuroimmunol.*, **1**, 137–40

53. Link, H., Norrby, E. and Olsson, J.-E. (1973). Immunoglobulins and measles antibodies in optic neuritis. *N. Engl. J. Med.*, **289**, 1103–7

54. Feasby, T. E. and Ebers, G. C. (1982). Risk of multiple sclerosis in isolated optic neuritis. *Can. J. Neurol. Sci.*, **9**, 269

55. Stendahl-Brodin, L. and Link, H. (1983). Optic neuritis: oligoclonal bands increase the risk of multiple sclerosis. *Acta Neurol. Scand.*, **67**, 301–4

56. Vandvik, B., Norrby, E. and Nordal, H. J. (1979). Optic neuritis: local synthesis in the central nervous system of oligoclonal antibodies to measles, mumps, rubella and herpes simplex viruses. *Acta Neurol. Scand.*, **60**, 204–13

57. Wells, J. V., Fudenberg, H. H. and Mackay, I. R. (1971). Relation of the human antibody response to flagellin to Gm genotype. *J. Immunol.*, **107**, 1505–11

58. Mackay, I. R., Wells, J. V. and Fudenberg, H. H. (1975). Correlation of Gm allotype, antibody response and mortality. *Clin. Immunol. Immunopathol.*, **3**, 408–11

59. Pandey, J. R., Goust, J.-M., Salier, J.-P. and Fudenberg, H. H. (1981). Immunoglobulin G heavy chain (Gm) allotypes in multiple sclerosis. *J. Clin. Invest.*, **67**, 1797–800

60. Propert, D. N., Bernard, C. C. A. and Simons, M. J. (1982). Gm allotypes and multiple sclerosis. *J. Immunogenet.*, **9**, 359–61

61. Francis, D. A., Brazier, D. M., Batchelor, J. R., McDonald, W. I., Downie, A. W. and Hern, J. E. C. (1986). Gm allotypes in multiple sclerosis: influence susceptibility in HLA-DQw1-positive patients from the north-east of Scotland. *Clin. Immunol. Immunopathol.*, **41**, 409–16

62. Blanc, M., Clanet, M., Berr, C., Dugoujon, J. M., Ruydavet, B., Ducos, S. J., Rascol, A. and Alpérovitch, A. (1986). Immunoglobulin allotypes in susceptibility ot multiple sclerosis. An epidemiological and genetic study in the Hautes-Pyrénées County of France. *J. Neurol. Sci.*, **75**, 1–5

63. Farid, N. R., Newton, R. M., Noel, E. P. and Marshall, W. H. (1977). Gm phenotypes in autoimmune thyroid disease. *J. Immunogenet.*, **4**, 429–32

64. Whittingham, S., Mathews, J. D., Schanfield, M. S., Tait, B. D. and Mackay, I. R. (1987). Interaction of HLA and Gm in autoimmune chronic active hepatitis. *Clin. Exp. Immunol.*, **43**, 80–6

65. Sandberg-Wollheim, M., Baird, L. G., Schanfield, M. S., Knoppers, M. H., Youker, K. and Tachovasky, T. G. (1984). Association of CSF IgG concentration and immunoglobulin allotype in multiple sclerosis and optic neuritis. *Clin. Immunol. Immunopathol.*, **31**, 212–21

66. Francis, D. A., Klouda, P. T., Brazier, D. M., Batchelor, J. R., McDonald, W. I. and Hern, J. E. C. (1988). Alpha-1-antitrypsin (PI) types in multiple sclerosis and lack of interaction with immunoglobulin (Gm) markers. *J. Immunogenet.*, **15**, 251–6.

67. Yam, P., Petz, L. D., Tourtellotte, W. W. and Ma, B. I. (1980). Measurement of complement components in cerebrospinal fluid by radioimmunoassay in patients with

multiple sclerosis. *Clin. Immunol. Immunopathol.*, **17**, 492–505
68. Compston, A. (1985). Immunological abnormalities in patients with optic neuritis. In Hess, R. F. and Plant, G. J. (eds.) *Optic Neuritis*, pp. 86–108. (Cambridge: Cambridge University Press)
69. Morgan, B. P., Campbell, A. K. and Compston, D. A. S. (1984). Terminal component of complement (C9) in cerebrospinal fluid of patients with multiple sclerosis. *Lancet*, **2**, 251–5
70. McMichael, A. J. and Sasazuki, T. (1977). A suppressor T cell in the human mixed lymphocyte reaction. *J. Exp. Med.*, **146**, 368–80
71. Bach, M. A., Tournier, E., Phan-Dinh-Tuy, F., Chatenoud, L. and Bach, J.-F. (1980). Deficit of suppressor T cells in active multiple sclerosis. *Lancet*, **2**, 1221–3
72. Reinherz, E. L., Weiner, H. L., Hauser, S. L., Cohen, J. A., Distaso, J. A. and Schlossman, S. F. (1980). Loss of suppressor T cells in active multiple sclerosis. *N. Engl. J. Med.*, **303**, 124–9
73. Compston, D. A. S. (1983). Lymphocyte subpopulations in patients with multiple sclerosis. *J. Neurol. Neurosurg. Psychiatry*, **46**, 105–14
74. Kastrukoff, L. F. and Paty, D. W. (1984). A serial study of peripheral blood T lymphocyte subsets in relapsing-remitting multiple sclerosis. *Ann. Neurol.*, **15**, 250–6
75. Rice, G. P. A., Finney, D., Braheny, S. L., Knobler, R. L., Sipe, J. C. and Oldstone, M. B. A. (1984). Disease activity markers in multiple sclerosis. Another look at suppressor cells defined by monoclonal antibodies OKT4, OKT5, and OKT8. *J. Neuroimmunol.*, **6**, 75–84
76. Kam-Hansen, S., Fryden, A. and Link, H. (1978). B and T lymphocytes in cerebrospinal fluid and blood in multiple sclerosis, optic neuritis, and mumps meningitis. *Acta Neurol. Scand.*, **58**, 95–103
77. Kam-Hansen, S., Rostrom, B. and Link, H. (1980). Active T cells and humoral immune variables in blood and cerebrospinal fluid in patients after acute unilateral idiopathic optic neuritis. *Acta Neurol. Scand.*, **61**, 298–305
78. Antel, J. P., Peebles, D. M., Reder, A. T. and Arnason, B. G. W. (1984). Analysis of T-regulator cell surface markers and functional properties in multiple sclerosis. *J. Neuroimmunol.*, **6**, 93–103
79. Cashman, N., Martin, C., Eizenbaum, J. F., Degos, J.-D. and Bach, M.-A. (1982). Monoclonal antibody-defined immunoregulatory cells in multiple sclerosis cerebrospinal fluid. *J. Clin. Invest.*, **70**, 387–92
80. Traugott, U. and Raine, C. S. (1984). Further lymphocyte characterisation in the central nervous system in multiple sclerosis. *Ann. N.Y. Acad. Sci.*, **436**, 163–78
81. Antel, J., Bania, M., Noronha, A. and Neely, S. (1986). Defective suppressor cell function mediated by T8+ cell lines from patients with progressive multiple sclerosis. *J. Immunol.*, **137**, 3436–9
82. Neighbour, P. A. (1984). Studies of interferon production and natural killing by lymphocytes from multiple sclerosis patients. *Ann. N.Y. Acad. Sci.*, **436**, 181–91
83. Sears, E., Tindall, R. and Zarnow, H. (1978). Active multiple sclerosis: enhanced computerized tomographic imaging of lesions and the effect of corticosteroids. *Arch. Neurol.*, **35**, 426–34
84. Harding, A. E., Radue, E. W. and Whiteley, A. W. (1978). Contrast enchanced lesions on computerised tomography in multiple sclerosis. *J. Neurol. Neurosurg. Psychiatry*, **41**, 754–8
85. Poser, C. (1980). Exacerbations, activity and progression in multiple sclerosis. *Arch. Neurol.*, **37**, 471–4
86. Dawson, J. W. (1916). The histology of disseminated sclerosis. *Trans. R. Soc. Edin.*, **50**, 517–40
87. Prineas, J. W. and Wright, R. G. (1978). Macrophages, lymphocytes and plasma cells in the perivascular compartment in chronic multiple sclerosis. *Lab. Invest.*, **38**, 409–21
88. Prineas, J. W. and Connell, F. (1978). The fine structure of chronically active multiple sclerosis plaques. *Neurology*, **28**, 68–75
89. Prineas, J. W., Kwon, E. E., Cho, E.-S. and Sharer, L. R. (1984). Continual breakdown and regeneration of myelin in progressive multiple sclerosis plaques. *Proc. N.Y. Acad. Sci.*, **436**, 11–32
90. Rucker, C. W. (1944). Sheathing of the retinal veins in multiple sclerosis. *Proc. Staff Mayo Clin.*, **19**, 176–8
91. Brinkman, C. J. J., Ter Laak, H. J., Hommes, O. R., Poppema, A. and Delmotte, P. (1982).

T lymphocyte sub-populations in multiple sclerosis lesions. *N. Engl. J. Med.*, **307**, 1644–5

92. Traugott, U., Reinherz, E. C. and Raine, C. (1983). Multiple sclerosis: distribution of T-cell subsets within active chronic lesions. *Science*, **219**, 308–10

93. Fontana, A., Fierz, W. and Wekerle, H. (1984). Astrocytes present myelin basic protein to encephalitogenic T cell lines. *Nature*, **307**, 273–6

94. Traugott, U. (1987). Multiple sclerosis: relevance of Class I and Class II MHC-expressing cells to lesion development. *J. Neuroimmunol.*, **16**, 283–302

95. Trotter, J. and Steinman, L. (1984). Homing of Lyt-2+ and Lyt-2– T cell subsets and lymphocytes to the central nervous system of mice with acute experimental allergic encephalomyelitis. *J. Immunol.*, **132**, 2919–23

96. Hafler, D. A. and Weiner, H. L. (1987). In vivo labelling of blood T cells: rapid traffic into cerebrospinal fluid in multiple sclerosis. *Ann. Neurol.*, **22**, 89–93

97. Tabira, T. and Sakai, K. (1987). Demyelination induced by T cell lines and clones specific for myelin basic protein in mice. *Lab. Invest.*, **56**, 518–25

98. Perry, L. L. and Bargaga, M. E. (1987). Kinetic and specificity of T and B cell responses in relapsing experimental allergic encephalomyelitis. *J. Immunol.*, **138**, 1434–41

99. Hafler, D. A., Benjamin, D. S., Burks, J. and Weiner, H. L. (1987). Myelin basic protein and proteolipid protein reactivity of brain and cerebrospinal fluid-derived T cell clones in multiple sclerosis and post-infectious encephalomyelitis. *J. Immunol.*, **139**, 89–102

100. Sedgwick, J., Brostoff, S. and Mason, D. (1987). Experimental allergic encephalomyelitis in the absence of a classical delayed-type hypersensitivity reaction. Severe paralytic disease correlates with the presence of interleukin-2 receptor positive cells infiltrating the central nervous system. *J. Exp. Med.*, **165**, 1058–75

101. Janzer, R. C. and Raff, M. C. (1987). Astrocytes induce blood brain barrier properties in endothelial cells. *Nature*, **325**, 253–7

102. Rawson, M. D., Liversedge, L. A. and Goldfarb, G. (1966). Treatment of acute retrobulbar neuritis with corticotrophin. *Lancet*, **2**, 1044–6

103. Rawson, M. D. and Liversedge, L. A. (1969). Treatment of retrobulbar neuritis with corticorophin. *Lancet*, **2**, 222

104. Bowden, A. N., Bowden, P. M. A., Friedman, A. J., Perkin, G. D. and Rose, F. C. (1974). A trial of corticotrophin gelatin injection in acute optic neuritis. *J. Neurol. Neurosurg. Psychiatry*, **37**, 869–73

105. Schmidt, D. (1983). Treatment of optic neuritis. *Bull. Soc. Belge Ophtal.*, **208**, 493–500

106. Panitch, H. S., Hirsch, R. L., Haley, A. S. and Johnson, K. P. (1987). Exacerbations of multiple sclerosis in patient treated with gamma interferon. *Lancet*, **2**, 893–5

107. Jacobs, L., Salazar, A. M., Herdon, R., Reese, P. A., Freeman, A., Jozefowicz, R., Cuetter, A., Husain, F., Smith, W. A., Ekes, R. and O'Malley, J. A. (1987). Intrathecally administered natural human fibroblast interferon reduces exacerbations of multiple sclerosis: results of a multicenter, double-blinded study. *Arch Neurol.*, **44**, 589–95

108. Bornstein, M. B., Miller, A. I., Teitelbaum, D., Arnon, R. and Sela, M. (1982). Multiple sclerosis: trial of a synthetic polypeptide. *Ann. Neurol.*, **11**, 317–9

8
Immunology of Ocular Tumours

A. GARNER and A. McCARTNEY

The discovery that some patients with cancer have circulating antibodies to their tumours aroused considerable interest, for not only did it afford a plausible explanation for the exceptional instances of spontaneous regression, but, more importantly, it was seen as a potential means of treatment, assuming that the response could be manipulated. Sadly, these initial hopes did not meet with immediate fulfilment and a wave of scepticism ensued to the extent that the immune response to neoplasms in general came to be regarded as an irrelevant epiphenomenon. More recently, however, the pendulum of opinion appears to be swinging back again on the basis that tumour-related antibodies, if not significantly cytotoxic in their own right, might serve as a device for the specific targeting of cytotoxic drugs to the tumour.

TUMOUR ANTIGENS

An immune response will be elicited in an immunocompetent host by any cell component that is new to the system. In the context of neoplasia, this presupposes the elaboration of a moiety by the tumour cells that is not recognized by the immune-surveillance mechanism. In theory, it may be located within the cell or on the cell surface. The former have not attracted much attention because, from a protective standpoint, they are likely to be of little consequence in that they are cut off from any specific antibodies or cell-mediated reaction by the cell membrane. Access on the part of the immune system is not hindered in this way, however, by antigens located on the cell surface and it is with such membrane-bound antigens that tumour immunology is principally concerned.

The immune response to tumour-generated cell-membrane-bound antigens is analogous in every way to allograft tissue rejection and, in consequence, it is appropriate that epitopes of this kind, which are not to be found in the non-neoplastic tissues, are referred to as tumour-specific transplantation

121

antigens. Some of the early studies in lower mammals concerning tumour-specific transplantation antigens invited criticism because inbred strains were not used, with the implication that the antigens responsible for immune rejection of grafted tumours could well have represented straightforward transplantation differences between heterogeneic animals. Nevertheless, subsequent experiments showed that similar rejection can be induced in inbred animal strains and even in the same animal if tumour cell implantation is attempted after extirpation of an identical primary tumour.

Tumour antigens capable of inducing rejection by the autologous host can be tumour-specific, to the extent that the responsible epitopes are totally new to be the host, or tumour-associated — representing either the renewed expression of genes normally operative only during fetal development before a competent immune surveillance mechanism has been established or the expression of increased amounts of antigens otherwise present in subliminal concentration.

Completely alien tumour antigens can be a feature of neoplasms induced by DNA viruses. Such viruses are integrated into the host genome and one of the consequences, should they provoke neoplastic transformation of the cell, is the expression of viral antigens at the cell surface. This means that tumours promoted by the same virus give rise to comparable neoantigen specificities irrespective of the host. Many of the best-studied virus-induced tumours have been experimentally promoted in lower mammals, but a naturally occurring example in humans is Burkitt's lymphoma involving Epstein–Barr virus infection.

Tumour antigens that may be present in subliminal amounts in the normal tissues probably include those attributable to carcinogenic chemical substances. Antigens of this kind have been studied extensively in experimentally induced tumours and shown to be peculiar to each individual tumour, so that cross-reactivity between histogenetically similar tumours induced by the same carcinogen is unusual. It has been speculated that the great diversity in antigen expression arises because the tumour-induced response is manifested in the variable regions of surface receptors involved in cellular interactions[1]. Such antigens are probably present on the surfaces of a few cells only under normal conditions and are able to escape the immune surveillance system. On the other hand, the massive increase in antigen associated with neoplastic clonal expansion of the relevant cell would reduce the chances of effecting such an escape.

The role of oncogenes in the induction of antigens with a capacity to induce tumour rejection also needs to be considered. Oncogenes appear to arise from naturally occurring genes, proto-oncogenes, that are provoked to undue levels of activity by the incorporation of viral DNA, by point mutations attributable to a variety of chemical and physical agencies, and possibly by a means as yet unidentified. Apart from their immediate role in deregulating the rate of cell proliferation, it is conceivable that the proteins encoded by the oncogenes will be antigenic and able to evoke an immune response. On the other hand, since it is probable that most, if not all, oncogene products represent quite minor alterations of normal proteins, it is to be expected that they will frequently fail to attract an immune response of consequence. This

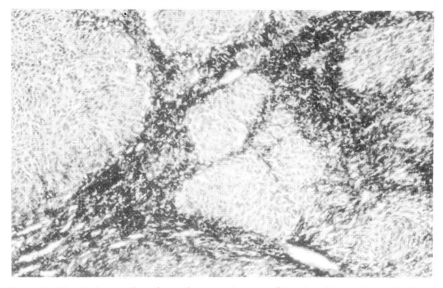

Figure 8.1 Histological section of a malignant melanoma of the choroid showing a spindle-cell tumour with lymphocytic infiltration seen as small, darkly-stained cells. (Haematoxylin and eosin, ×135)

may explain the failure of the majority of cancers to stimulate an effective rejection response.

There are also those antigens that, whilst they are an expression of the neoplastic state, are not typically associated with a rejection response. Among such tumour-associated antigens are those normally expressed during maturation of the fetus *in utero* but not thereafter. Known as oncofetal antigens they may reappear in later life as a feature of certain types of tumour. Two of the better known oncofetal antigens are carcinoembryonic antigen in conjunction with adenocarcinomas of the colon and α-fetoprotein in patients with hepatocellular carcinoma. Rarely, they may be linked with antibody formation by the host, although there is no good evidence that they have any effect on tumour behaviour. Another group of tumour-associated antigens occurs as a manifestation of cell differentiation but, being a component of healthy non-neoplastic cells of the same histogenesis, they do not evince an immune response in the autologous host. They can, nevertheless, provide useful 'markers' for tumour diagnosis, given the availability of antisera raised in a xenogeneic situation.

IMMUNE RESPONSE TO NEOPLASIA

The first inklings that malignant tumours might evoke an immune reaction that would operate against the tumour came from clinical experience and circumstantial histological observations (Figure 8.1). Spontaneous regression, although rare, has been reliably attested in histologically confirmed tumours[2] and metastases have been known to regress after excision of the primary lesion[3]. Lymphocytic infiltration of carcinoma of the breast has also been reported to correlate with prognosis following surgery[4]. Furthermore, immunodeficient individuals, whether their condition be primary or secondary to drug-induced immunosuppression, have been reported to run an enhanced risk of developing certain types of cancer owing, possibly, to failure of the immune-surveillance mechanism to recognize virus-transformed target cells[5].

B-cell response

Despite the prevailing view that antibodies are subordinate to cell-mediated responses in any modifying effect the immune system might have on tumour behaviour[6], interest in the B-cell response has been revived by recognition of the potential value of using tumour-specific antibodies as a homing device for the delivery of cytotoxic agents.

In a study of cutaneous melanoma, Lewis *et al.*[7] were able to show that the serum of a patient contained antibodies able to inhibit the growth of cells from that patient's tumour grown in tissue culture. Sera from allogeneic melanoma patients had a lesser effect. Evidence of a significant effect *in vivo*, whether in respect of skin melanoma or other malignancies, is sparse. The antibodies responsible for the *in vitro* inhibition appear to be mainly of the IgG class and to act in one of two ways. Complement fixation may be involved[8] or, alternatively, the effect may be indirect through antibody-dependent cell-mediated cytotoxicity wherein the Fc regions of IgG2a and IgG3 antibodies combine with receptor sites on phagocytic cells. Allied to conventional antigen–antibody combination at the target cell surface, this serves to bring activated cytotoxic cells into contact with the tumour[9,10].

T-cell response

It is generally considered that cellular responses are more important than antibody as effectors of tumour rejection and, in view of the high degree of specificity of the process, it is reasonable to suppose that T cells are implicated. The precise role of the T-cell subsets and their interactions with other cellular and humoral factors is, however, not entirely clear.

T cells have been shown to exercise tumour cytotoxicity *in vitro* in respect of autologous but not allogeneic cancers[11], and the further finding that these responses may be matched by an improved prognosis suggests that there could be an *in vivo* counterpart[12].

Whilst it might be expected that cytotoxic T cells would be prominent in tumour rejection, the situation appears to be more complex in that helper CD4+ T cells are probably the key element in the overall regulation of the cellular response[11]. There is the further possibility that these CD4+ T cells can function as cytotoxic effector cells[13]. Tumour cells can be induced to express Class II major histocompatibility complex (MHC) antigens by lymphokines such as interferon-γ. These cells then become targets for activated LD4+ T cells, which can kill cells in a different manner from that of the Class I restricted CD8+ T cells. Secretion of lymphotoxin by the CD4+ T cells is thought to be one of the lymphokines involved in the cytotoxic mechanism[14]. There is also evidence that the CD4+ T cells can act against tumour cells in an indirect manner through the secretion of lymphokines, especially lymphotoxin[14].

Natural killer cells

NK cells are a type of lymphocyte, characterized morphologically by their large size and slightly granular cytoplasm, that can lyse tumour cells independently of MHC expression. Experiments in rats have shown that reducing the number of NK cells in the circulating blood impairs the capacity to reject mammary carcinoma cells[15]. NK-cell activity can be augmented by interleukin-2 and interferon and, possibly, other lymphokines released in the course of specific tumour-oriented T-cell responses. The extent to which NK cells are a significant part of the immune reponse to human tumours is uncertain and, while the therapeutic administration of interferons may initially boost NK cell activity, the effect is likely to be short-lived[16].

Lymphokine-activated killer cells

LAK cells are yet another type of lymphocyte which exhibit cytolytic activity when stimulated by interleukin-2 liberated by activated T cells as a result of tumour sensitization[17]. They have no effect on normal cells and can lyse tumour cells that are unaffected by NK cells. Beneficial effects have been claimed in patients with metastatic cancer following the injection of LAK cells in the presence of interleukin-2.

Macrophages

Macrophages that have been activated by T-cell-derived lymphokines, especially interferon-γ, may also exhibit selective toxic effects on tumour cells. The effect is mediated by the release of lytic enzymes, oxygen radical formation and the production of tumour necrosis factor, a lymphokine which often works synergistically with interferon-γ[6]. Conversely, macrophages can also serve to suppress NK cell and T cell activity and there is some evidence that they may even stimulate tumour cell growth[18]. Correspondingly, the overall clinical effect of macrophages on tumour behaviour is far from clear.

EVASION OF IMMUNE TUMOUR RESPONSES

Cancers in general, including those affecting humans, evoke an immune response that has the potential to destroy the tumours. Conversely, there is an enchanced predisposition for immunodeficient individuals to develop cancer. In the face of these two complementary observations, it is relevant to investigate the seeming ineffectiveness of the observed immune rejection process in the vast majority of cancer patients. A number of possibilities merit consideration.

Imbalance between tumour growth rate and immune response

For the immune system to be stimulated, it is necessary to have a minimal level of antigenic stimulation and even when sensitization does eventually occur it may initially lag behind the tumour expansion in quantitative terms. In this way, a tumour might become established before there is an appreciable immune rejection capability or, as it is sometimes expressed, the tumour 'sneaks through'[19,20].

Blocking antibodies

It has been shown experimentally that antibodies may be present that are not only unable to mediate cell death because they fail to fix complement but that may interfere with the T-cell response directed against the tumour[21]. An early belief that the blocking was due to prior combination of the antibody with antigens on the tumour cell surface later gave way when it was shown that immune complexes involving free (soluble) antigenic determinants are implicated. How this impairs T-cell cytolytic activity has yet to be resolved[22].

Immune suppression

It has long been recognized that patients with advanced cancers commonly show non-specific depression of cell-mediated immunity as measured by the cutaneous response to a variety of antigens[23]. More recently, experiments in mice have shown that whereas the initial reaction to tumours is expressed in terms of enchanced cell-mediated activity, this is followed by a negative suppressor cell response[24]. Interesting, and possibly of therapeutic significance, is the finding that removal of the primary tumour early in the course of the disease can reverse the suppressor effect. Whether the latter observation is the explanation of the re-emergence of antibody after surgery remains to be seen[7].

IMMUNOLOGICAL MODULATION OF THE CAPACITY FOR TUMOUR METASTASIS

Information concerning the way in which immunological processes may affect the ability of a tumour to disseminate has come from a study of mice inoculated with cloned syngeneic carcinoma cells, some of which had a high metastatic potential while others had little or no such capacity despite originating from the same tumour[25]. It was found that the immune response, as measured by the generation of T-lymphocyte-mediated cytotoxicity, was inversely related to the metastatic capacity of the inoculum.

Subsequently, the difference in immunogenicity was shown to be a reflection of the ratio of two separate type 1 MHC antigens on the surface of the tumour cells, the expression of which is determined by a specific oncogene. Whether these observations are applicable to the human situation has yet to be determined, but, if they are, they suggest that it is before the metastasizing cells reach their destination, particularly as they enter the lymphatics and bloodstream, that the disseminating cells are most vulnerable to immunological attack.

CLINICAL APPLICATIONS OF TUMOUR IMMUNE RESPONSES

It is disappointing that although most, and possibly all, tumours provoke an immune response, the vast majority of established lesions appear to be little affected by it. Whether the incidence of cancer and perhaps more specifically of distinct metastases would be higher in the absence of an immune response, whilst distinctly possible, is hard to assess. As yet, attempts to augment the rejection potential of the tumour rejection reaction using adjuvants and a range of cytokines aimed at activating cellular mechanisms towards the cellular effectors have not met with conspicuous success. In part, this may be due to ignorance of the relative importance of the different cellular components of the rejection phenomenon in humans as opposed to animal models, so that attempts at modulation are misdirected. In part it may also be that any step to increase the wanted response has to compete with the spontaneous suppression of downregulation of the immune system that is commonly observed.

Nevertheless, several practical and potentially beneficial applications of the anti-tumour immune response have been identified.

Cytotoxic drug delivery using monoclonal antibodies

The hybridoma technique for fusing myeloma cells and splenocytes from mice previously immunized with tumour-cell components means that it is possible to produce large amounts of highly specific antibody *in vitro*. Cloning of the hybridoma cells offers the further prospect that antibodies to specific tumour determinants can be generated exclusively. The antigens concerned tend to be tumour-related, rather than tumour-specific, since the subsequent antibodies commonly cross-react *in vitro* with other tumours of similar histogenesis, and appear to be mostly oncofetal or differentiation antigens. Whilst the antibodies to which they give rise do not promote tumour rejection, it is possible they can, nevertheless, be manipulated for chemotherapeutic purposes. Thus, if they are conjugated with a cytotoxic substance and then injected into the circulating blood they will ideally serve as a homing device to deliver the drug or other agent to the tumour in preference to other tissues. In this way, harmful effects on the non-cancerous tissues will be kept to a minimum whilst achieving effective dosage of the tumour.

Certain lectins, of which ricin is a prime example, are highly cytotoxic by virtue of their ability to interfere with ribosome function and can be linked with tumour-associated antibodies as anticancer agents[26]. Such combinations have been found to be effective in experimental tumour models and some initial reports of their use in the management of human tumours are encouraging[26,27]. A number of radionuclides and other cytotoxic drugs have also been conjugated with monoclonal tumour antibodies. A potential limitation of this mode of selective cytotoxic agent delivery is the risk that the patients will develop antibodies to the monoclonal antibody (anti-idiotype), since the latter is a product of murine splenocytes and as such is xenogeneic to the host. There is, however, the intriguing prospect that such anti-idiotype antibodies could themselves be tagged with a cytotoxic agent to increase the level of drug delivery to the tumour[26,27].

Clinical diagnosis

Monoclonal antibodies, which will cross-react with other tumours of similar histogenesis, can also be used as an aid to clinical diagnosis by tagging them with radioactive tracer elements[27]. As the labelled antibodies aggregate within the tumour they can be detected by scintillation recording techniques and the lesion can be both identified and delineated[28].

Histopathological diagnosis

Specific cell types can be identified in histological sections of tumours using antibodies raised against determinants peculiar to or highly characteristic of those cells. For instance, antibodies to glial fibrillary acidic protein are useful in the identification of tumours of astrocytic origin and antibodies to S-100 protein react with cells derived from the neural crest[29]. Evidence of antigen–antibody interaction is commonly demonstrated by conjugating the antibodies either with fluorescein or with horse-radish peroxidase, the latter being particularly valuable in the immunostaining of conventional paraffin sections. The precision of tumour diagnosis in terms of histogenesis can be greatly enhanced in this way.

The second half of this chapter will deal with three important types of tumour that are problems in ophthalmological practice. Melanomas of the choroid, while much rarer than their counterparts in skin, are the most common intraocular tumours to be seen in clinical ophthalmology, although autopsy results suggest that metastatic carcinomas from lung or breast may have a higher incidence. Retinoblastoma is a childhood tumour that can be inherited as an autosomal dominant disease, when both eyes are affected; it also occurs as a sporadic mutation, once in 30000 births and persons with unilateral disease may subsequently be capable of transmission of the disease to their offspring if the mutation occurs early in embryogenesis. In this country retinoblastoma is usually detected in its intraocular phase, but is capable in some instances of invading through the corneoscleral shell into the orbit and meninges.

The third group of tumours to be discussed will be those presenting as orbital tumours, especially those of lymphoid origin.

MHC CLASS ANTIGENS AND TUMOURS OF THE EYE

The major histocompatibility complex antigens (MHC), or human leukocyte antigens (HLA) in man, are divided into three classes[30]. Class I antigens are found on the surface of almost all nucleated cells in the body, and in the eye have been demonstrated by some workers[31] on the epithelium and external basement membrane of the ciliary body, on the anterior border of the iris and on vascular endothelial cells within the iris and choroid, whilst others have disputed their expression on normal uveal cells[32]. Changes in the expression of Class II antigens may result in greater oncogenicity as a result of diminished T-cell surveillance.

Autoimmune disease is known to be associated with increased expressivity of HLA DR3 and to a lesser extent HLA DR4: in these diseases there is a genetic predisposition that allows an uncontrolled proliferation of clones of lymphoid cells, capable of destroying cells or tissues that they fail to recognize as self. Cells displaying the 'inappropriate' HLA antigens are treated as if they were of foreign extraction. Similarly, in tumours the uncontrolled clonal growth phase may also be associated with anomalous expression of Class II antigens on proliferating cells and this may attract the attention of the immunoregulatory system with a consequent T-cell response.

No Class II expression is seen on normal melanocytes of the skin or eye. Equally, Class II expression is not seen in naevi, although some expression of Class I MHC has been observed in these benign proliferations of melano- cytes[33]. Melanomas of the skin express both Class I and II, with Class II antigen expression increasing with depth of the tumour and also in clumps of tumour cells that have metastasized elsewhere in the body. Class I and II antigen expression is particularly evident in tumours surrounded by a brisk chronic inflammatory cell response[34]. However, aberrant Class II antigen expression does not seem to parallel other indicators of a poor prognosis such as increasing diameter or scleral invasion. Transplantation of tumours expressing Class II antigens into athymic nude mice results in rapid loss of the ability to express HLA DR antigens[35] but retention of HLA DP and DQ and other melanoma-associated antigens. Melanoma cells expressing Class II antigens may therefore act directly as antigen-presenting cells *in vitro* without the need for the passage of information through conventional antigen- presenting cells such as macrophages or B cells, now known to be the commonest antigen-presenting cells elsewhere in the body[36]. B cells are not observed in ocular melanomas, even in those infiltrated with large numbers of lymphocytes[37]. Malignant melanomas expressing HLA DR are more effective at autologous lymphocytic activation in culture and the activated autologous lymphocytes are cytotoxic from the initiating tumour. Interestingly though, cells grown from metastases from these tumours may lose the ability to stimulate autologous lymphocyte production whilst retaining Class II expression, which may even be enhanced[38]. Class II MHC antigens can stimulate allogeneic lymphocytes in over 60% of cases, with further augmentation by interferon. Similar Class II antigen aberrant expression enhanceable by interferon-γ is seen in retinoblastomas, including the cultured cell line Y79, in lymphomas and leukaemias.

Since not all retinoblastoma cells express Class II antigen activity, it has been suggested that expression may play a part in differentiation, since in moderately differentiated tumours between 65% and 95% of cells express the antigens, whereas in poorly differentiated tumours only 8–10% of cells carry

HLA DR[39]. Class I MHC expression is even rarer, moderately differentiated tumours having 5–10% positive cells and undifferentiated tumours less than 2%.

The loss of Class II MHC expression as the tumour becomes progressively less well differentiated is echoed in uveal melanomas, no HLA DR activity being detectable in an investigation of epithelioid or necrotic tumours, whilst spindle B or mixed tumours showed widespread positivity[37]. This study also investigated the nature of the lymphoid response excited by the tumours. No B-cell infiltration was seen at all, but epithelioid melanomas had more than 50 T cells per high-power field (HPF) of both helper (CD4) and cytotoxic-suppressor (CD8) type. Mixed or spindle B tumours had fewer than 5 T cells per HPF. Twenty to thirty macrophages per HPF were present in all tumours but natural killer cells were only seen in necrotic tumours. Another extensive review[40] of the numbers of lymphocytes present in over one thousand melanomas on the files of the Armed Forces Institute of Pathology showed that melanomas with increased lymphoid infiltrates (more than 100 lymphocytes per 20 HPF), had a reduction in 15-year survival from 62% to 42% ($p = 0.00001$) and this remained significantly important even after known factors such as tumour size, position, cell type and the presence of necrosis, scleral or orbital invasion were taken into account.

Patients with metastatic melanoma terminally have reduced T-cell rosetting with diminished immunocompetence, whereas patients without metastatic disease but with melanomas that pierce the sclera (or primary conjunctival melanoma) have evidence of an accentuation of their immune responses, both humoral and cell-mediated[41]. Many of these patients with heightened responses subsequently died of metastatic disease. Patients with melanomas have increased circulating B and T cells, both CD4 and CD8 subtypes. The augmentation of the lymphoid response at this overtly invasive stage of the tumour's history may be a reflection of the overriding of the protective influence, in terms of diminished delayed-type hypersensitivity (DTH), conferred by the anterior chamber-associated immune deviation (ACAID) first described in mice[42]. In mice, ACAID requires an intact spleen for its elaboration. Removal of the spleen allows delayed-type hypersensitivity reactions to occur even in tumours that have not breached the sclera. Splenectomy does not alter the immune response in man, since DTH is regulated by the thymus without the spleen. ACAID in man is circumvented by acquisition of local antigen-presenting capacity by cells such as tumour cells or Langerhans cells in the cornea that do not normally present or by induction through the conjunctival lymphoid circuit system.

Metastasis of intraocular tumours to the lung can be augmented experimentally through activation of peritoneal macrophages by thioglycol-late[43] and by enucleation, or even external pressure to the globe, coupled to T-cell deficiency or the use of antisialo-GMI serum to diminish NK cell function[44]. It is paradoxical, therefore, that increased localized T-cell response in tumours is linked to a poor prognosis, whilst an absent T-cell response is even less advantageous. Experimentally, the use of interferon-γ to enhance the NK response suppresses metastasis. Tumour necrosis is often associated with a poor prognosis in choroidal melanomas but a prolonged investigation of the effect of apparent spontaneously necrotic rejection foci in cutaneous melanomas showed that no advantage or disadvantage is conferred by such foci in terms of survival.

SPONTANEOUS REGRESSION

In patients presenting with metastatic cutaneous melanoma, spontaneous regression of the primary tumour is thought to have occurred in up to 12% of the cases[45]. Spontaneous regression of metastatic disease is much less common, probably in the region of 0.25% and only 40% of these regressed tumours are fully cured. Spontaneous regression of ocular melanomas is also uncommon but well documented in 3.8% of phthisical eyes that unexpectedly are found to contain tumour[46].

Spontaneous regression of retinoblastomas (leaving aside the cases that would now be diagnosed as retinocytomas and which consist only of benign differentiated cells), is associated with calcification and phthisis. Calcification is so common that it is used as a diagnostic criterion in ultrasound or X-ray diagnosis, but complete regression is sufficiently rare for only 50 cases to have been recorded by 1977[45]. Some authors have rejected the idea of immunologically-mediated regression[48] and think that the process depends on vascular insufficiency, especially following occlusion of the central retinal artery. They cite those cases of bilateral disease in which there is phthisis in one eye and rampantly invasive tumour in the other, implying that immunologically mediated rejection cannot have occurred. This apparent anomaly could, however, be due to heterogeneous expression of tumour antigenicity at different times, varying with the degree of differentiation in tumours, even within the same patient. Similar mechanisms may also account for the varying immunological response in primary and secondary tumours, where display of different antigenic profiles may result in differing responses and variable amounts of tumour necrosis. Antigen expression can vary in metastases in the same patient and even within the same tumour deposits[49].

MELANOMA

Melanomas of the eye develop in the conjunctiva, iris, ciliary body and choroid. Naevi and malignant melanoma of the uvea arise from melanocytes of neural crest origin. They usually contain the pigment melanin, synthesized from tyrosine via DOPA (3,4-dihydroxyphenylalanine) and dopaquinone, using tyrosinase as a catalyst. Although apparently amelanotic tumours are well recognized, they usually contain small amounts of melanin, but metastatic secondary tumours may lose the ability to secrete melanin. The pigment is found in intracytoplasmic organelles — melanosomes. The cells of the pigmented epithelia of the iris, ciliary body and retina contain melanin, but within melanosomes that are much larger, whilst the cells are derived not from the neural crest but from the outgrowth of the neuroectoderm that forms the optic vesicle. The neural crest-derived melanocytes and the tumours that arise from them are therefore more like those found in the skin and much of the research into ocular melanomas shadows that into cutaneous melanomas. Many of the antigens that have been studied are shared between the two groups of tumours and some of the cell products seen in cultured melanocytes, from both ocular and skin tumours, reflect the cells' migratory characteristics in fetal life. Migrating melanocytes secrete plasminogen activator and fibronectin to smooth their passage between tissues and use vimentin cytoplasmic intermediate filaments to move; all of these primitive cell products have been described in cultured melanocytes.

Genetic instability, with sequential selections of clones of variant subpopulations of cells, is common in tumours[50], but melanocytes seem especially vulnerable. Some melanocyte populations appear inherently unstable, such as those in the dysplastic naevus syndrome. Some can be made unstable by exogenous factors such as inappropriate amounts of UV light for the degree of natural pigmentation. This probably explains the raised incidence of melanomas in the pale-skinned Scots-Irish, especially migrants to Australia and possibly the increased incidence of melanomas of the choroid in those with pale irides. Heavy racial pigmentation of the skin and uvea acts as a protection against mutation in the melanocytic DNA as well as in other surrounding cells, such as those of the basal layer of the skin, so that cutaneous melanomas (and basal cell carcinomas) are uncommon in blacks.

The progression from normality through naevi to dysplasia of the naevi and melanoma should ideally be marked through changing and definable antigenicity in the cell membrane or cytoplasm. Unfortunately, most melanoma-associated antigens are quantitatively rather than qualitatively different in tumour cells[51] when compared with their normal counterparts. The search for such melanoma-associated antigens (MAAs) has yielded at least 65 antigens capable of definition by monoclonal antibodies. Many of these are not specific to melanocytes or melanomas, being widely distributed on different cells and tissues throughout the body. Some are associated with fetal life and expression in the adult is therefore inappropriate. Others are restricted to expression on melanocytes, their tumours or other neuroecto-dermal or primitive neuroectodermal derivatives and some are so restrictive that they only recognize homologous tumour cells. These last may be of value in defining and treating metastatic foci within one patient but clearly have no wide applicability. The three groups of melanoma-associated antigens discussed below are those defining origin from melanocytes, the melanocytic lineage markers, some of which are structural or constitutional; others that are thought to represent different stages of melanocytic evolution, referred to as stage-specific markers; and a third group that are intracytoplasmic markers, often used in immunohistochemical identification of tumours.

Melanocyte lineage markers

Of the markers that recognize and define cells of the melanocyte lineage, the monoclonal antibody (Mab) R24[52], which was the most restrictive of a panel of Mabs used in an assessment of 25 uveal melanomas (although widely demonstrable in cutaneous melanomas), is an IgG3 antibody recognizing a ganglioside GD3. This glycolipid is demonstrable in the cytoplasm of other neuroectodermal structures at or near the Golgi apparatus but is only found as a cell surface marker in melanocytes, where it is carried on the cell external membrane or on the adhesion plaque. Unlike other melanoma-associated antigens (MAAs), including Class II antigens, it is not removable by the action of the chelating agent EDTA[53]. GD3 mediates detachment and aggregation of cells, and when shed in culture it enhances the growth of other tumours, such as murine lymphomas. GD3 also regulates T-cell-mediated immunity, as shown by inhibition of mitogen-induced lymphocytic attraction *in vitro*. Its derivative GD2[54], thought to be the oncofetal antigen described by Irie[55], is produced after catalysis by N-acetylgalactosaminyl transferase. GD2 promotes the adhesion of melanoma cells to solid substrates by increasing their stickiness and also promotes metastasis by tumour shedding[56]. The Mab R24 has been used clinically with success and the treated necrotic tumours show infiltration by lymphocytes and degranulating mast cells rather than polymorphonuclear leukocytes[10].

The other widely recognized marker of melanocytic lineage is a high-molecular-weight proteoglycan, similar to chondroitin sulphate[49], that is membrane-associated but not bound and is easily shed in culture and extractable by mild dissociation. Both the GD3 and the proteoglycan may be examples of inappropriate retention or expression of a material that is then able to be detected on surveillance as a 'foreign' surface antigen. Both are variably expressed, usually as reciprocals of one another, with GD3 being prominent on the most differentiated melanocytic tumours.

Stage-specific markers for melanomas

One of the most interesting concepts to emerge in the study of MAAs is that of sequential expression of different MAAs identifying different stages of evolution of the tumour, in contrast to the constitutional markers such as GD3 and proteoglycan[57]. These have been serologically typed and divided into early, intermediate and late markers. Melanomas expressing undifferentiated or primitive characteristics have early markers and are epithelioid and unpigmented, with low levels of tyrosinase activity. Those expressing intermediate-type markers resemble fetal and newborn melanocytes[51] with a spindled or bipolar shape, whilst those melanocytic cells with late markers are of adult-type, polydendritic, heavily pigmented and have high levels of tyrosinase activity and do not form tumours. Some discrepancy between the levels of HLA DR positivity in these cultured epithelioid melanomas and the surgically resected tumours examined by Smith *et al.*[37] is possibly accounted for by the observation that cultured cells often express a wider and more primitive range of products than their tissue counterparts owing to lack of physiological controls.

Another widely investigated antigen expressed by most melanomas is the antigen described as p97[49], to which at least 20 different monoclonal antibodies have been raised, and which has five epitopes: it is a sialoprotein varying in quantity from 500 000 molecules per cell down to 20 000, at which level it is difficult to detect, so that the tumour may be erroneously described as 'negative'. The molecule has great structural similarities to transferrin and is capable of binding iron; it is coded for on the same part of chromosome 3 as both transferrin and its receptor, the latter being thought to be identical to B lym, a known oncogene. p97 may also act as a growth factor by binding iron and conferring an evolutional advantage on cells expressing it. The wide variation in expression of MAAs[58] probably follows loss of genetic material, something that may occur in any somatic cell but that is more easily observed in cells with a high mitotic rate. Dracopoli's[59] group used DNA probes recognizing restriction fragment-length polymorphisms to establish that loss of genetic material occurred from eight different chromosomes in a group of 24 cutaneous melanomas and that the frequency of loss was between 8% and 67%, reflecting the dissimilarity of tumours from different hosts and even different sites as clonal selection occurs.

This contrasts with the more restricted loss of genetic material in the inherited form of retinoblastoma, which seems to occur only on chromosome 13 and may account for the more limited phenotypic variation and expression of markers that seems to occur.

Immunohistochemistry of melanomas

Immunohistochemical markers have been used to identify cells in tissue sections and improve the accuracy of diagnosis. In the immunodiagnosis of ocular tumours, one of the most consistently useful markers is S100[60], an acidic protein found as a dimer with three possible isomers; it binds calcium and was thought initially to be glial-specific. S100 was subsequently demonstrated in Schwann cells and melanocytes and their malignant counterparts, although there is loss of positivity in up to 50% of malignant schwannomas. S100 protein is found in the cytoplasm and the nucleoplasm and may also be expressed on the membrane of the cells. Expression may be dependent on the cell cycle and this may account for the variability of staining within a given tumour and for differences in expression between tumours. Almost all cutaneous melanomas contain S100, but in ocular melanomas the antigen was only demonstrable[61] on 33 tumours in a series of 60, being most heavily expressed in areas of high mitotic rate and heavy pigmentation. The nerve fibres within the tumour were also positive, as were the perivascular glial cells within the retina. The antigenicity of retinal glial cells and Müller's cells within the retina has been hotly disputed, but there does seem to be some species variation and some of the anomalous results may arise as a result of using bovine brain to produce most commercially available antisera. Bovine brain is deficient in the α subunit of S100 and therefore cells with the $\alpha\alpha$ isomeric structure $S100a_0$ expressed may not be seen as positive[62]. Elevated levels of S100 within the vitreous (but not the aqueous) of eyes containing choroidal melanomas have been demonstrated by radioimmunoassay[63]. Another marker used in the immunodiagnosis of intraocular tumours is the γ subtype of neurone-specific enolase, again originally thought to be limited in its expression to the CNS but subsequently demonstrated elsewhere. In the same series of 60 choroidal melanomas, it was seen in necrotic and epithelioid areas of the tumours where there was more macrophage infiltration. The

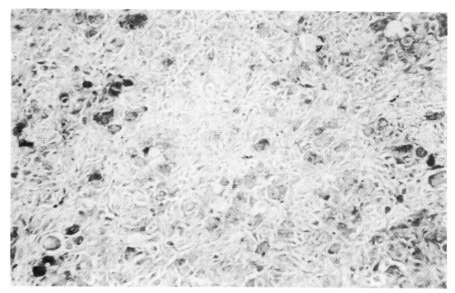

Figure 8.2 Epithelioid cells in mixed choroidal malignant melanoma staining positively with antibodies to PGP 9.5. (Immunohistochemistry using naphthal AS-MX phosphoric acid and fast red TR Salt, ×315)

expression of neurone-specific enolase was the only marker to be correlated with a poor prognosis.

Protein gene product 9.5 (PGP9.5) is also a soluble protein found in neurones and also identified in melanocytic lesions. This marker is more common than S100 in ocular melanomas, although the distribution is different in that the marker is most often seen close to the entry site of nerves into the tumour in cells clustered around the nerve twiglets, which are themselves positive[64] (Figure 8.2).

RETINOBLASTOMA

The gritty white masses of tumour found within the eye containing retinoblastoma are thought to have developed from the precursors of the photoreceptor cells or possibly from primitive neuroectoderm before any differentiation. Most of the inherited tumours are discovered early in life and almost all retinoblastomas are diagnosed before the age of 3 years[65].

The tumour consists of primitive cells, sometimes arranged in the form of rosettes, and in rare instances further differentiation towards photoreceptors is seen in structures called fleurettes. Necrosis, followed by calcification, is extremely common.

Antigenicity of retinoblastomas

Cell-mediated immunity to retinoblastomas is demonstrable by skin testing[66], but the nature of the antigens exciting the reaction is uncertain. The introduction of monoclonal antibodies has removed the hazards to interpretation caused by background staining and non-specific polyclonal reactions and the range of antigens studied has been broadened. Light microscopy and electron microscopy tend to favour the hypothesis that the tumour derives from cells already differentiated towards photoreceptor elements rather than from undifferentiated bipotential neuroectodermal precursor cells capable of expressing neuronal or astrocytic features. Some workers have reported separate foci and glial elements not apparently arising as a reaction to the tumour on histology, and retinoblastoma lines are said to have produced glial differentiation in culture[67].

Antigens demonstrated immunohistochemically in retinoblastomas include the rod outer segment marker rhodopsin[68], which is seen as a surface marker forming a halo around cells, and S antigen, which is seen within the cytoplasm. S antigen, also known to localize to rod outer segments, can be demonstrated on Flexner–Wintersteiner rosettes and fleurettes, the better-differentiated photoreceptor-like areas. Interestingly, in tumours where these areas are present, S antigen will also be found on cells in the undifferentiated areas. If there are no differentiated areas, no S-antigen can be shown[69], which suggests that there may indeed be two phenotypically different types of retinoblastoma, those with some photoreceptor differentiation and those that may be more primitive neuroectodermal or glial tumours. Other elements can be demonstrated immunohistochemically.

Amacrine cell markers such as substance P and preproencephalin A have been described in retinoblastoma, as well as the documented cross-reaction of somatostatin with amacrine cells. Also present are insulin and insulin receptor, thought to be localized on to neurones or Müller cells. A triplet neurofilament protein of 200 kDa, which is thought to be a neurocytoskeletal element, can also be demonstrated[70], as can the intraretinal binding protein (IRBP) that has been synthesized by Y79 cells in culture[71].

Neurone-specific enolase, of the γ sub-type, thought to be found in photoreceptors and neurones rather than astrocytic cells[72], is seen in retinoblastomas and is extractable from the tumour as well as from the aqueous humour. The pattern of staining observed by different groups of workers varies, some seeing staining of rosettes and fleurettes, others describing the staining in more undifferentiated areas. Glial fibrillary acidic protein (GFAP) positive astrocytes (see below) have been well described in many papers, most seem to be reactive components rather than neoplastic, with the characteristic pattern of staining showing positive cells around blood vessels, in necrotic areas or radiating out from unaffected areas to form a capsule around the tumour rather than forming independent masses, although this has also been described. The intermediate filament vimentin has also been shown in cells within the tumour but is again thought to represent a reaction to the tumour[73].

HLA Class II antigens inducible by retinoic acid and enhanced by interferon have been described in cultured cells, but the oncofetal antigens CEA and AFP, although raised in the sera of some patients with retinoblastoma, have not been demonstrable in the tumour *in vivo* or *in vitro*.

ORBITAL TUMOURS

The majority of orbital tumours present with proptosis, optic nerve compression, limitation of ocular movements and variable amounts of pain. Metastatic tumours are not uncommon and can be confused clinically and radiologically with primary tumours. The problem of inflammatory lesions, the so-called 'pseudotumours', and the overlap with lymphoid neoplasia are also discussed below.

Immunohistochemistry and orbital tumours

The diagnosis of soft-tissue tumours within the orbit is greatly facilitated by the use of immunohistochemical markers of intermediate filaments. A wide range of dependable monoclonal antibodies has allowed greater confidence in diagnosing these tumours and lessened the need for electron microscopy. Although soft tissue tumours are rare, comprising only 1% of all human malignancies[74] they often present diagnostic problems. This problem is accentuated within the orbit, since up to 35% of metastatic tumours of the orbit are from unknown or occult sites and may mimic primary tumours.

Cytoplasmic filaments

Cytoplasmic filaments are divisible into three categories[75] — (1) large microtubules 20–25 nm in diameter, which are monomers of tubulin that do not vary between cell types; (2) thin filaments, 5–6 nm in diameter, that can be divided into those associated with muscle and those not, by staining with antiactin monoclonal antibodies; and (3) the group known as intermediate filaments, which define the cytoskeletal components. This third group of 10 nm diameter filaments is formed by polypeptide subunits polymerized into fibrils in the cytoplasm to form bundles or meshworks. They are cell-type restricted so that the marker vimentin, although found in all fetal cells, in the adult is seen in vascular endothelial cells and fibroblasts but can also be expressed by tumours such as melanomas and rarely by astrocytes. Muscle can be recognized immunohistochemically by the use of antibodies to desmin. This expression is an extremely useful marker for the undifferentiated embryonic rhabdomyosarcomas of the orbit seen in children (Figure 8.3).

High- and low-molecular-weight cytokeratins can be demonstrated singly or in combination. Squamous epithelium expresses high-molecular-weight cytokeratin and simple cuboidal epithelium has low-molecular-weight cytokeratin, whilst ductal epithelia express both together. Neurones, as has already been discussed, contain neurofilaments, and neurofilament marker has been shown in the rare nasal tumour that may affect the orbit, the aesthesioneuroblastoma.

Glial fibrillary acidic protein (GFAP) is expressed by astrocytes and developing but not mature oligodendroglia and Bergman radial glia and has been described in tumours arising from the lacrimal gland[76].

Interestingly, these pleomorphic adenomas also express two other intermediate-filament markers simultaneously. It is rare for tumours to express more than one marker and no explanation for the apparently

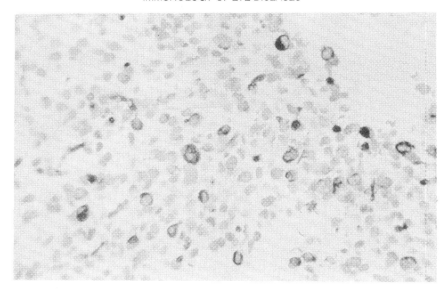

Figure 8.3 Embryonal rhabdomyosarcoma immunostained with monoclonal antibody to desmin. (Immunoperoxidase PAP-DAB, ×338)

anomalous expression of GFAP on cells other than glia has been found; the other two markers are vimentin and a cytokeratin. This latter combination has been associated with tissues where epithelial and myoeithelial cells coexist, as in the ductal elements of the lacrimal gland.

In addition to the markers of intermediate filaments, monoclonal and polyclonal antisera to other markers may be useful in tumour diagnosis. These include labelled antibodies to myoglobin, actin and myosin to demonstrate muscle origin, and Factor VIII, which stains endothelial cells and megakaryocytes and enzyme markers such as alpha 1 trypsin and chymotrypsin that may help to identify tumours composed of histiocytes. Also widely used are lymphocyte markers, often in combination with the cytokeratin markers such as CAM 5.2, to establish whether a poorly differentiated lesion is a carcinoma or lymphoma.

Orbital lymphomas and lymphoproliferative disease

Although in the rest of the body almost a third of lymphomas will be of Hodgkin's type, the disease hardly ever occurs in the orbit, where almost all orbital lymphomas are of B-cell lineage although rare spread from the post-nasal space of a T-cell lymphoma (which is much commoner in the Japanese), may be envisaged. The malignant lymphomas form one end of the spectrum of lymphoproliferative disease of the orbit. The orbit is a unique site containing mesodermal and neuroectodermal derivatives without any lymphatic drainage behind the orbital septum. There is little normal lymphoid tissue, other than scattered lymphocytes and plasma cells in the stroma of the lacrimal gland, the numbers of which increase with advancing age, presumably as a response to prolonged exposure to a wide range of antigens. Lymphoid follicles are not usually seen.

Lymphomas of the non-Hodgkin type have been divided into low-grade, intermediate and high-grade types. Those categorized as low-grade are of small cell type, resembling normal lymphocytes with and without plasmacytoid features and the follicular lymphomas. The intermediate types tend to be more diffuse and the cells are generally larger, whilst the highest-grade lymphomas are composed of large cells, either primitive centre cells, the lymphoblastic type, or ill-formed plasma-cell precursors, the immunoblastic-plasmacytoid group. Burkitt's lymphoma is also regarded as a high-grade lymphoma[77].

Lymphoproliferative disease is a continuum, starting with frankly hyper-plastic lesions in which well-defined follicles, containing developing cells and histiocytes, are seen mixed with other inflammatory cells such as eosinophils. There is lymphocytic maturation to plasma cells. These lesions show both κ and λ light-chain positivity and are described as polyclonal. In particular, the plasma cells are polyclonal for light-chain expression. Clinically, the lesions are usually painful and may progress to fibrosis. There is some overlap between these reactive processes and conditions in which there may be an element of autoimmunity, such as dysthyroid eye disease and posterior scleritis.

The next group in the range is the polyclonal but morphologically banal group of small lymphocytic cell proliferations, with a paucity of other cell types, that have been described as indeterminate lymphoid proliferations but in which current follicle formation is not seen. This group merges imperceptibly with those lesions not exhibiting any light-chain markers and presumed incipient lymphomas that show disturbance of the κ–λ ratio with light-chain restriction and monoclonality. At the far end of the scale are those tumours that are so poorly differentiated that they are lymphoblastic in nature and do not display light chains and other tumours that are plasmacytoid in nature with a monoclonal immunoglobulin that is usually IgA. Large-cell immunoblastic tumours are seen that may not show monoclonality. Reactions to the lymphoid proliferation may be T-cell-mediated with recruitment of a polyclonal B-cell infiltrate that can complicate interpretation of light-chain staining, especially at the phase of early clonal proliferation. Recent research (Hyjek, McCartney, Isaacson, unpublished observations) has shown evidence of erstwhile follicles, marked by the EN11 antiserum, in a group of lymphomas with light-chain restriction, underscor-ing the evolution of neoplastic lesions from presumed reactive lesions with progressive loss of control of the proliferating cells until a monoclonal population becomes predominant. Control of this proliferation may be within the T-cell regulatory system and the number of T cells within a lymphopro-liferative lesion within the orbit has been used to aid diagnosis[78].

Although, traditionally, non-steroid responsive lymphoproliferative dis-ease has been treated with low-dose radiotherapy on the assumption that there is little tendency for it to spread outside the orbit, prolonged follow-up has shown that this is not always the case. Bilateral and recurrent disease is well recognized and in the group of monoclonal (light-chain restricted) lesions examined by Hyjek *et al.*, a disturbing tendency for the lesions to re-emerge in the para-aortic nodes was seen. This is somewhat unlike the distribution of lymphomas from sites thought to be similar in type, i.e. the mucosa-associated tumours found in the salivary gland, the thyroid and lung (also referred to as mantle-zone lymphomas), from which bone-marrow spread is commoner. The association with autoimmune disease in these sites, especially the thyroid and salivary gland, also bears comparison with orbital lymphomas, especially those within the lacrimal gland, although myoepithelial islands are not a common finding.

References

1. Flood, P. M., DeLeo, A. B., Old, L. J. and Gershon, R. K. (1983). Relation of cell surface antigens on methylcholanthrene induced fibrosarcomas to immunoglobulin heavy chain complex variable region linked T cell interaction molecules. *Proc. Natl. Acad. Sci. USA*, **80**, 1683–7

2. Everson, T. C. and Cole, W. H. (1966). *Spontaneous Regression of Cancer: A Study and Abstract of Reports in the World Medical Literature and of Personal Communications Concerning Spontaneous Regression of Malignant Disease.* (Philadelphia: W. B. Saunders)

3. Jenkins, G. D. (1959). Regression of pulmonary metastasis following nephrectomy for hypernephroma: eight year follow-up. *J. Urol.*, **82**, 37–40

4. Cutler, S. J., Black, M. M., Mork, J., Harvei, S., and Freeman, S. (1969). Further observations on prognostic factors in cancer of the female breast. *Cancer*, **24**, 653–67

5. Purtilo, D. T. (1988). Opportunistic cancers in patients with immunodeficiency syndromes. *Arch. Pathol. Lab. Med.*, **111**, 1123–9

6. Robins, R. A. (1987). Basic tumour immunology. In Byers, V. S. and Baldwin, R. W. (eds.) *Immunology of Malignant Diseases*, pp. 1–28. (Lancaster: MTP)

7. Lewis, M. G., Ikonopisir, R. L., Nairn, R. C., Phillips, T. M., Fairley, G. H., Bodenham, D. C. and Alexander, P. (1969). Tumour-specific antibodies in human malignant melanoma and their relationship to the extent of the disease. *Br. Med. J.*, **3**, 547–52

8. Capone, P. M., Papsidero, L. D., Groghan, G. A. and Chu, T. M. (1983). Experimental tumoricidal effects of monoclonal antibody against solid breast tumors. *Proc. Natl. Acad. Sci. USA*, **80**, 7328–32

9. Adams, D. O., Hall, T., Steplewski, Z. and Koprowski, H. (1984). Tumors undergoing rejection induced by monoclonal antibodies of the IgA2a isotype contain increased numbers of macrophages activated for a distinct form of antibody dependent cytolysis. *Proc. Natl. Acad. Sci, USA*, **81**, 3506–10

10. Houghton, A. N., Mintzer, D., Cordon-Carlo, S., Welt, S., Fleigel, B., Vadhan, Carswell, E., Melamed, M. R., Oettgen, H. F. and Old, L. J. (1985). Mouse monoclonal IgG3 antibody detecting GD3 ganglioside: a phase I trial in patients with malignant melanoma. *Proc. Natl. Acad. Sci. USA*, **82**, 1242–6

11. Vose, B. M. (1987). Immunomodulating agents. In Byers, B. S. and Baldwin, R. W. (eds.) *Immunology of Malignant Diseases*, pp. 70–82. (Lancaster: MTP)

12. Vanky, F., Klein, E., Willems, J., Brook, K., Ivert, T., Peterffy, A., Nilsonne, V., Kreicbergs, A. and Aparisi, T. (1986). Lysis of autologous tumor cells by blood lymphocytes tested at the time of surgery: correlation with the postsurgical course. *Cancer Immunol. Immunother.*, **21**, 69–76

13. Janeway, C. A., Bottomly, K., Babich, J., Conrad, P., Conzen, S., Jones, B., Kaye, J., Katz, M., McVay, L., Murphy, D. P. and Tite, J. (1984). Quantitative variation in Ia expression plays a central role in immune regulation. *Immunol. Today*, **5**, 99–105

14. Gray, P. W., Aggarawal, B. B., Benton, C. V., Bringman, T. S., Henzel, W. J., Jarrett, J. A., Leung, D. W., Moffat, B., Ng, P., Svedersky, L. P., Palladino, M. A. and Nedwin, G. (1984). Cloning and expression of cDNA for human lymphotoxin, a lymphokine with tumour necrosis activity. *Nature*, **312**, 721–4

15. Barlozzari, T., Leonhardt, J., Wiltrout, R. H., Herberman, R. B. and Reynolds, C. W. (1985). Direct evidence for the role of LGL in the inhibition of experimental tumour

metastasis. *J. Immunol.*, **134**, 2783–9

16. Maluish, A. E., Ortaldo, J. R., Conlon, J. C., Sherwin, S. A., Leavitt, R., Strong, D. M., Wernick, P., Oldham, R. K. and Herberman, R. B. (1983). Depression of natural killer cell cytotoxicity after in vivo administration of recombinant leukocyte interferon. *J. Immunol.*, **131**, 503–7

17. Rosenberg, S. A. (1985). Lymphokine activated killer cells: a new approach to immunotherapy of cancer. *J. Natl. Cancer Inst.*, **75**, 595–603

18. Evans, R. (1978). Macrophage requirement for growth of a murine fibrosarcoma. *Br. J. Cancer*, **37**, 1086–9

19. Old, L. J., Boyse, E. A., Clarke, D. A. and Carswell, F. A. (1962). Antigenic properties of chemically induced tumors. *Ann. N.Y. Acad. Sci.*, **101**, 80–106

20. DeBoer, R. J., Hogeweg, P., Dullens, H. F. J., DeWeger, R. A. and DenOtter, W. (1985). Macrophage T lymphocyte interactions in the antitumor immune response: a mathematical model. *J. Immunol.*, **134**, 2748–58

21. Hellstrom, I., Sjogren, H. O., Warner, G. and Hellstrom, K. E. (1971). Blocking of cell-mediated tumor immunity by sera from patients with growing neoplasms. *Int. J. Cancer*, **7**, 226–37

22. Hellstrom, K. E., Hellstrom, I. and Nepom, J. T. (1978). Specific blocking factors — are they important? *Biochim. Biophys. Acta*, **473**, 121–48

23. Harris, J. E. and Sinkovics, J. G. (1970). *The Immunology of Malignant Disease.* (St. Louis: Mosby)

24. North, R. J. (1985). Down-regulation of the antitumour immune response. *Adv. Cancer Res.*, **45**, 1–43

25. Eisenbach, L., Kushtai, G., Plaksin, D. and Feldman, M. (1986). MHC genes and oncogenes controlling the metastatic phenotype of tumour cells. *Cancer Rev.*, **5**, 1–18

26. Baldwin, R. W. and Byers, V. S. (1987). Monoclonal antibody targeting of cytotoxic agents for cancer therapy. In Byers, V. S. and Baldwin, R. W. (eds.) *Immunology of Malignant Disease*, pp. 44–54. (Lancaster: MTP)

27. Goldenberg, D. M. (1988). Targeting of cancer with radiolabeled antibodies: prospects for imaging and therapy. *Arch. Pathol. Lab. Med.*, **112**, 580–7

28. Pimm, M. V. (1987). Immunoscintigraphy: tumour detection with radiolabelled antitumour monoclonal antibodies. In Byers, V. S. and Baldwin, R. W. (eds.) *Immunology of Malignant Disease*, pp. 21–43. (Lancaster: MTP)

29. Kahn, H. J., Marks, A., Thorn, H. and Baumal, R. (1983). Role of antibody to S-100 protein in diagnostic pathology. *Am. J. Clin. Pathol.*, **79**, 341–7

30. Jager, M. J., van der Pol, J. P., de Wolff-Rouendaal, D., de Jong, P. V. T. M. and Ruiter, D. J. (1988). Decreased expression of HLA Class II antigens on human uveal melanoma cells after in vivo X-ray irradiation. *Am. J. Ophthalmol.*, **105**, 78–86

31. Bakker, M. and Kijlstra, A. (1985). The expression of HLA antigens in the human anterior uvea. *Curr. Eye Res.*, **4**, 599–604

32. Abi-Hanna, D., Wakefield, D. and Watkins, S. (1988). HLA antigens in ocular tissues. I. In vivo expression in human eyes. *Transplantation*, **45**, 610–13

33. Ruiter, D. J., Bhan, A. N., Harrist, T. J., Sober, A. J. and Mihm, M. C. (1982). Major histocompatibility antigens and mononuclear inflammatory infiltrate in benign nevomelanocytic proliferations and malignant melanoma. *J. Immunol.*, **129**, 2808–15

34. Taramelli, D., Fossati, G., Mazzochi, A., Delia, D., Ferrone, S. and Parmiani, G. (1986). Classes I & II HLA and melanoma-associated antigen expression and modulation on melanoma cells isolated from primary and metastatic lesions. *Cancer Res.*, **46**, 433–9

35. van der Brink, M. E. M., van Muijen, C. T., Guyt, C. J., Schrier, P. I. and Ruiter, D. J. (1986). Suppression of HLA-Class II expression in human melanoma cells xenografted to nude mice. *J. Pathol.*, **149**, 237A

36. Abbas, A. K. (1987). Cellular reactions in the immune response. The roles of B lymphocytes and interleukin-4. *Am. J. Pathol.*, **129**, 26–33

37. Smith, M. D., Liggett, P. E. and Rao, N. A. (1988). Immunohistochemical characterisation of lymphoid infiltration in human choroidal melanomas. *Invest. Ophthalmol. Vis. Sci.* (ARVO Abst.), **29**, 365

38. Fossati, G., Taramelli, D., Balsari, A., Bodganovich, S., Andreola, A. and Parmiani, G. (1984). Primary but not metastatic human melanomas expressing DR antigens stimulate

autologous lymphocytes. *Int. J. Cancer*, **33**, 591–7

39. Detrick, B., Chader, G., Katz, N. and Rodrigues, M. (1988). Evaluation of Class II antigen expression and cellular differentiation in retinoblastoma. *Invest. Ophthalmol. Vis. Sci.* (ARVO Abst.) **29**, 340

40. De La Cruz, P. O., Specht, C. S. and McLean, I. W. (1988). Lymphocytic infiltration of uveal melanoma. *Invest. Ophthalmol. Vis. Sci.* (ARVO Abst.), **29**, 365

41. Cochran, A. J., Foulds, W. S., Damato, B. E., Trope, G. E., Morrison, L. and Lee, W. R. (1985). Assessment of immunological techniques in the diagnosis and prognosis of ocular malignant melanoma. *Br. J. Ophthalmol.*, **69**, 117–26

42. Niederkorn, J. Y. and Streilein, J. W. (1983). Alloantigens placed into the anterior chamber of the eye induce specific suppression of delayed-type hypersensitivity but normal cytotoxic T lymphocyte and helper T lymphocyte responses. *J. Immunol.*, **131**, 2670–4

43. Gorelik, E., Wiltrout, R. H., Copeland, D. and Herberman, R. B. (1985). Modulation of formation of tumour metastases by peritoneal macrophages elicited by various agents. *Cancer Immunol. Immunother.*, **19**, 35–42

44. Niederkorn, J. Y. (1984). Enucleation in consort with immunologic impairment promotes metastasis of intraocular melanomas in mice. *Invest. Ophthalmol. Vis. Sci.*, **25**, 1080–6

45. Bodurtha, A. J., Berkelhammer, J., Kim, Y. H., Laucius, J. F. and Mastrangelo, M. J. (1976). A clinical histological and immunologic study of a case of malignant melanoma undergoing spontaneous remission. *Cancer*, **37**, 735–42

46. Makley, T. T. and Teed, R. W. (1958). Unsuspected intraocular malignant melanomas. *Arch. Ophthalmol.*, **60**, 475–8

47. Khodadoust, A. A., Roozitalab, H. M., Smith, R. E. and Green, W. R. (1977). Spontaneous regression of retinoblastoma. *Surv. Ophthalmol.*, **21**, 467–78

48. Zimmerman, L. E. (1984). Retinoblastoma and retinocytoma. In Spencer, W. H. (ed.) *Ophthalmic Pathology, An Atlas and Textbook*, Vol. II, pp. 1292–351. (Philadelphia: W. B. Saunders)

49. Hellstrom, K. E. and Hellstrom, I. (1985). Monoclonal antimelanoma antibodies and their possible clinical use. In Baldwin, R. W. and Byers, V. S. (eds.) *Monoclonal Antibodies for Cancer Detection and Therapy*, pp. 17–51. (London: Academic Press)

50. Klein, G. and Klein, E. (1985). Evolution of tumours and the impact of molecular oncology. *Nature*, **315**, 190–5

51. Houghton, A. N., Cordon-Cardo, C. and Eisinger, M. (1986). Differentiation antigens of melanoma and melanocytes. *Int. Rev. Exp. Pathol.*, **28**, 217–48

52. Dippold, W. G., Lloyd, K. D., Li, L. T. C., Ikeda, H., Oettgen, H. F. and Old, L. J. (1980). Cell surface antigens of human malignant melanoma. Definition of six antigenic systems with monoclonal antibodies. *Proc. Natl. Acad. Sci. USA*, **77**, 6114–18

53. Cheresh, D. A., Harper, J. R., Schultz, G. and Reisfeld, R. (1984). Localisation of the gangliosides GD_2 and GD_3 in adhesion plaques and on the surface of human melanoma cells. *Proc. Natl. Acad. Sci. USA*, **81**, 5767–71

54. Thurin, J., Thurin, M., Herlyn, M., Elder, D. E., Steplenski, Z., Clark, W. H. and Koprowski, H. (1986). GD_2 ganglioside biosynthesis is a distinct biochemical event in human melanoma tumor progression. *FEBS*, **208**, 17–22

55. Irie, R. F., Sze, L. and Saxton, R. E. (1982). Human antibody to OFA-1, a tumour antigen produced in vitro by EBV transformed human B lymphoid cell lines. *Proc. Natl. Acad. Sci. USA*, **79**, 5666–70

56. Ladisch, S., Kitada, S. and Hays, E. F. (1987). Gangliosides shed by tumor cells enhance tumor formation in mice. *J. Clin. Invest.*, **79**, 1879–82

57. Brocker, E.-B., Suter, L., Bruggen, J., Ruiter, D. J., Macher, E. and Sorg, C. (1985). Phenotypic dynamics of tumor progression in human malignant melanomas. *Int. J. Cancer*, **36**, 29–35

58. van der Pol, J. P., Jager, M. J., de Wolff-Rouendaal, D., Ringens, P. J., Vernegoor, C. and Ruiter, D. J. Heterogeneous expression of melanoma associated antigens in uveal melanomas. *Curr. Eye Res.*, **6**, 757–65

59. Dracopoli, N. C., Houghton, A. N. and Old, L. J. (1985). Loss of polymorphic restriction fragments in malignant melanoma: implications for tumour heterogenicity. *Proc. Natl. Acad. Sci. USA*, **82**, 1470–4

60. Cochran, A. J., Holland, G. N., Wen, D. R., Herschman, H. R., Lee, W. R., Foos, R. Y. and

Straatsma, B. R. (1983). Detection of cytoplasmic S100 protein in primary and metastatic intraocular melanomas. *Invest. Ophthalmol. Vis. Sci.*, **24**, 1153–5

61. Williams, R. A., Rode, J., Dhillon, A. P., Charlton, I. G. and McCartney A. (1987). P.G.P. 9.5, S100 protein and neurone specific enolase in ocular melanomas. *J. Pathol.*, **152**, 195A

62. Kivela, T. and Tarkkanen, A. (1986). S100 protein in retinoblastoma revisited. *Acta Ophthalmol.*, **64**, 664–73

63. Cochran, A. J., Holland, G. N., Saxton, R. E., Damato, B. E., Foulds, W. R., Herschman, R., Foos, R. Y., Straatsma, B. R. and Lee, W. R. (1988). Detection and quantification of S100 protein in ocular tissue and fluids from patients with intraocular melanoma. *Br. J. Ophthalmol.*, **72**, 874–9

64. McCartney, A. C. E., Johns, J., Rode, J., Dhillon, A. P., Wilson, P. O. G., Charlton, I. G., Williams, R. A., Dhillon, B. and Hungerford, J. (1989). Recent advances in the histopathological study of ocular melanomas. *Eye* (In press)

65. McCartney, A. C. E., Olver, J. M., Kingston, J. E. and Hungerford, J. L. (1988). Forty years of retinoblastoma; into the fifth age. *Eye*, Suppl. 2, S13–18

66. Char, D. H. and Heberman, R. B. (1974). Cutaneous delayed hypersensitivity responses to standard recall antigens and crude membrane extracts of retinoblastoma tissue culture cells. *Am. J. Ophthalmol.*, **78**, 40–4

67. Kyritsis, A. P., Tsokos, M., Triche, T. J. and Chader, G. J. (1984). Retinoblastoma — origin from a primitive neuroectodermal cell? *Nature*, **307**, 471–3

68. Donoso, L. A., Hamm, H., Dietzschold, B., Augsberger, J. J., Shields, J. A. and Arbizo, V. (1986). Rhodopsin and retinoblastoma. A monoclonal antibody histopathologic study. *Arch. Ophthalmol.*, **104**, 111–13

69. Mirshahi, M., Boucheix, C., Dhermy, P., Haye, C. and Faure, J.-P. (1986). Expression of the photoreceptor-specific S antigen in human retinoblastoma. *Cancer*, **57**, 1497–500

70. Rickman, D., Murphree, A. L. and Brecha, N. (1987). Neurofilament immunoreactivity in retinoblastoma. *Invest. Ophthalmol. Vis. Sci.* (ARVO Abst.), **28**, 24

71. Campbell, M. A., Lish, A., Karras, P., Wiggert, B., Lee, L., Hayden, B. and Chader, G. J. (1988). IRBP synthesis by Y 79 cells induction by butyrate and suppression by laminin. *Invest. Ophthalmol. Vis. Sci.* (ARVO Abst.), **29**, 341

72. Kivela, T. (1986). Neurone specific enolase in retinoblastoma. An immunohistochemical study. *Acta Ophthalmol.*, **64**, 19–25

73. Kivela, T., Tarkkanen, A. and Virtanen, I. (1986). Intermediate filaments in the human retina and retinoblastoma. An immunohistochemical study of vimentin, glial fibrillary acidic protein and neurofilaments. *Invest. Ophthalmol. Vis. Sci.*, **27**, 1075–84

74. DuBoulay, C. E. H. (1985). Immunohistochemistry of soft tissue tumours: a review. *J. Pathol.*, **146**, 77–94

75. Gown, A. M. and Vogel, A. M. (1985). Monoclonal antibodies to intermediate filament proteins III. Analysis of tumors. *Am. J. Clin. Pathol.*, **84**, 413–24

76. Orcutt, J. C., Ree, H. M. J., Gown, A. M. and Lindquist, T. D. (1987). Diagnosis of orbital and periorbital tumours; use of monoclonal antibodies to cytoplasmic antigens (intermediate filaments). *Ophthalm. Plast. Reconstruct. Surg.*, **3**, 159–78

77. Rosenberg, S. (1982). National Cancer Institute-sponsored study of classification of non-Hodgkin's lymphomas. Summary and description of a working formulation for clinical usage. *Cancer*, **49**, 2112–35

78. Knowles, D. M. and Jakobiec, F. A. (1981). Quantitative determination of T cells in ocular lymphoid infiltration. An indirect method for distinguishing between pseudolymphomas and malignant lymphomas. *Arch. Ophthalmol.*, **99**, 309–16

9
Immune Disorders with Ocular Involvement

K. FAIRBURN and D. A. ISENBERG

INTRODUCTION

Autoimmune disorders represent a spectrum of disease but may be broadly divided into those that affect many organs or systems and those which are organ-specific. In this chapter we will review the immunological features of the 'classical' autoimmune diseases and of some of the closely allied rheumatological and vasculitic disorders, such as ankylosing spondylitis, Reiter's syndrome and Behçet's disease, in which ocular involvement may be a feature.

AUTOIMMUNE RHEUMATIC DISEASES

Sjögren's syndrome

Henrik Sjögren, a Swedish ophthalmologist, first emphasized the association association of dry eyes, dry mouth and rheumatoid arthritis. Sjögren's syndrome (SS) is now recognized as one of the commonest autoimmune rheumatic diseases (ARDs), second only to rheumatoid arthritis (RA). It results from inflammatory infiltration and destruction of exocrine glands, in particular the salivary and lacrimal glands. Primary SS is the combination of keratoconjuctivitis sicca (KCS) and xerostomia. Primary extraglandular SS includes those patients who, in addition, manifest systemic features. Secondary SS defines patients with an additional recognizable ARD.

Patients with KCS complain of gritty discomfort and foreign body sensations, photophobia and redness of the eye. Superadded infection, often with staphylococcus, may exacerbate these symptoms. Complications affecting the eye include corneal ulceration, vascularization and, rarely, perforation.

Systemic features include a nodular vasculitis with purpura and hyperviscosity syndromes related to hyperglobulinaemia. Fifty per cent of patients with SS have RA and 20% have another ARD, most frequently systemic lupus erythematosus (SLE) or scleroderma[1]. Conversely about 20–25% of patients with RA and SLE have secondary SS. Other associations include polymyositis (15%), primary biliary cirrhosis (50–100%), chronic active hepatitis (50%), autoimmune thyroid disease, pernicious anaemia, renal tubular acidosis, glomerulonephritis and lymphoproliferative disorders.

The immunopathology of Sjögren's syndrome

The histological features in the minor lip gland biospy are the same as those in the lacrimal and salivary glands, namely lymphocytic infiltration ranging from discrete foci to dense, almost confluent infiltration with destruction of acini and ducts[2,3].

The major immunological findings in the salivary glands of patients with Sjögren's syndrome are the presence of HLA Class II (DR) antigens on glandular epithelial cells, often accompanied by the presence of interferon-γ; many T-helper cells expressing activation markers; activated B cells; the production of monoclonal immunoglobulins and the relative absence of NK cells[4]. There are also many plasma cells whose cytoplasm contains IgA. Horsfall et al.[5] have demonstrated that anti-La idiotypes may be found within these plasma cells.

In the peripheral blood of patients with Sjögren's syndrome, polyclonal hypergammaglobulinaemia is present and 60% or more of patients have rheumatoid factors and antibodies which are Ro and La. In addition, monoclonal immunoglobulins may be found and there is deficient interleukin-2 (IL-2) production and decreased NK cell function. It is tempting to believe that the persistence of viruses such as Epstein–Barr virus and cytomegalovirus in the salivary glands may be the trigger that sets the disease in motion[6]. It is of course important to remember that EBV is commonly found in the salivary epithelium of healthy people. Thus, any response giving rise to Sjögren's syndrome is clearly inappropriate. Assuming, however, that the viral trigger is important, the steps outlined in Figure 9.1 may indeed be an accurate reflection of what is happening in these patients.

A strong association between HLA DR3 and SS has been demonstrated, implying a strong genetic component in the aetiology of this condition.

Systemic lupus erythematosus

Systemic lupus erythematosus (SLE) is a chronic inflammatory disorder predominantly affecting young women. Multiple organ systems are involved resulting in a wide range of clinical manifestations with accompanying immunological abnormalities.

Ocular manifestations of SLE include erythema and oedema of the eyelids, blepharitis, conjunctivitis, episcleritis, scleritis, Sjögren's syndrome and retinopathy[7].

Retinopathy is considered rare in SLE patients[8]. Clinically observed retinal lesions include cotton-wool spots (9–24%) and flame haemorrhages (10%). Less common are retinal arteritis and phlebitis, which may result in occlusion

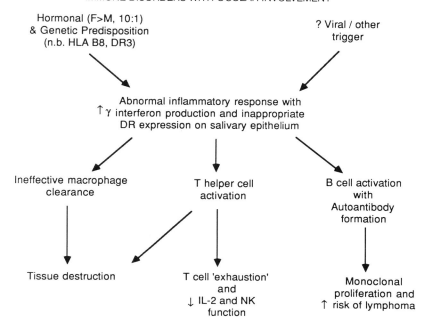

Figure 9.1 Suggested pathway leading to the clinical expression of Sjögren's syndrome

of the affected vessels[9]. Swelling of the optic disc can result from inflammation of the vessels within the optic nerve. Occlusion of the vessels may occur, resulting in ischaemic optic neuropathy[10]. The prognosis for recovery in the latter is poor. Retinal detachment occurs rarely and most often terminally[11]. Cytoid bodies (cotton-wool spots) may occur and represent infarctions of the nerve-fibre layer. These may occur independently of renal involvement. Microvascular abnormalities may be detected with fluorescein angiography in the absence of clinical evidence of retinal disease[12]. Retinopathy is associated with disease activity, cerebral involvement and is a marker of poor prognosis for survival[13]. This is confirmed by the observations of retinopathy being more common in the pre-steroid era and occurring in patients whose disease activity is not well controlled.

Aetiology

Lupus is relatively common among females. It occurs predominantly in women between the ages of 20 and 30 with a female:male ratio of 9:1. There is a varying prevalence between countries and racial groups. One in 250 Black females develops lupus in contrast to 1:4000 caucasian females[14,15]. Genetic factors considered important in the aetiology of SLE include the association with major histocompatibility antigens (MHCs) HLA A1, B8 and DR3. There is also a 2–4% prevalence rate in first-degree relatives with a high

Table 9.1 Prevalence of autoantibodies in systemic lupus erythematosus

Anti-ds DNA	50–90%
Anti-ss DNA	≃ 70%
Anti-histones	≃ 70%
Anti-poly (ADP-ribose)	70%
Anti-cardiolipin	20–50%
Anti-RNP	20–35%
Anti-thyroglobulin	Up to 35%
Anti-thyroid microsomes	Up to 35%
Anti-Ro	30%
Rheumatoid factor	≃ 25%
Anti-Sm	25% (in USA)
	5% (in Europe)
Anti-La	15%

concordance rate (about 70%) between identical twins. In contrast, the concordance rate amongst dizygotic twins is about 12%[16].

Environmental factors that may play a role include UV light and a wide range of drugs, e.g. hydralazine and procainamide, dietary factors and possibly viruses.

Immunopathology of SLE

SLE is often thought of as the classic autoimmune disease, with high levels of circulating immune complexes that deposit in a variety of tissues, activating complement with ensuing tissue damage. However, the early notions that these complexes would consist mainly of DNA bound to anti-DNA antibodies have not been borne out. In fact, the actual constituents of most of these complexes remain obscure. In addition, although there is polyclonal, or probably oligoclonal[17] B-cell expansion, whether this is truly antigen-driven, dependent on excessive T-cell help, or arises *de novo* is uncertain.

An impressive array of autoantibodies is detectable in lupus patients. These include antibodies binding to DNA, the phospholipids, Ro, La, Sm, RNP, and antibodies binding to the surface of a variety of cells including red cells and platelets[4]. The approximate frequency with which these antibodies are found in lupus patients is shown in Table 9.1. It has, however, been very difficult to demonstrate the presence of any of these antibodies, or indeed their antigens, in the immune complexes detectable in lupus patients. Whatever the stimulus for the production of these autoantibodies, it is possible that they may be binding to antigens already present or possibly 'planted' in the relevant tissues.

Defects in virtually every component of the immune repertoire have been demonstrated in lupus patients. A summary of the major cellular defects is shown in Figure 9.2. It has also become evident that defects in cytokine metabolism may be playing a role in lupus. For example, impaired IL-2 production and responsiveness have been found in lupus patients, as have elevated levels of interferon-α[18].

T cell compartment

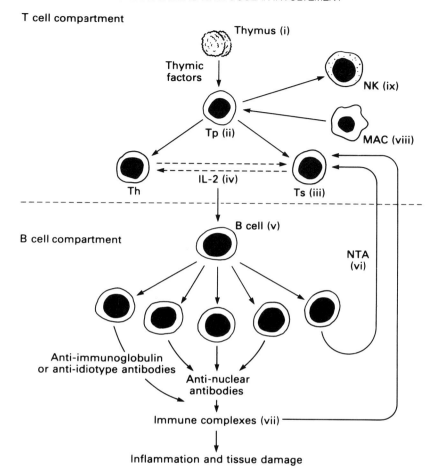

Figure 9.2 An outline of the major cellular defects in systemic lupus erythematosus. *T-cell compartment:* (i) defective thymus processing, decreased production of thymic factors; (ii) decreased numbers and dysfunction of post-thymic precursor cells (Tp); (iii) defective suppressor T cells (Ts) fail to regulate the B lymphocyte compartment, although induction of antibodies continues owing to excess T-helper (Th) cell function; (iv) impaired IL-2 secretion and unresponsiveness causes further imbalance in the T-cell populations. *B-cell compartment:* (v) a primary B-cell defect exists; (vi) secretion of antilymphocyte or natural thymocytotoxic antibody (NTA) amplifies regulatory disorder; (vii) immune complexes may further impair suppressor T-cell function, as well as causing tissue damage. *Accessory cells:* (viii) macrophages may contribute to the autoimmune process. (Reproduced from Morrow, W. J. W. *et al.* (1983). *Lancet,* **2,** 206, with permission.)

Exhaustive studies of segments within the hypervariable regions of anti-DNA antibodies, designated idiotypes, have provided notable insights into the immunoregulatory disturbances present in lupus patients. One common or public idiotype designated 16/6 has been identified in the serum of over half of the lupus patients studied and in over 40% of the kidney biopsies taken from lupus patients[19]. Most interestingly, mRNA sequencing of this idiotype has shown that its sequence is identical to that of a germline gene designated VH 26[20]. Furthermore, it has been shown that the 16/6 idiotype is not confined to antibodies that bind to DNA but is also present on antibodies that bind the Klebsiella polysaccharide antigen K30[19]. It would thus appear that a common idiotype that may well be involved in the pathogenesis of SLE is actually germline encoded! Presumably it has been preserved because, under normal circumstances, it is part of antibodies concerned with host defence. However, in lupus patients, production of the idiotype is 'subverted' and large quantities of anti-DNA antibodies carrying this idiotype are produced. In support of the view that this idiotype may indeed be pathogenic, a recent study by Mendelovic et al.[21] has demonstrated that immunization of healthy mice with an antibody bearing this 16/6 idiotype led, after 4 months, to the development of a lupus-like disease with alopecia, leukopenia and a wide range of autoantibodies and glomerulonephritis. Independent confirmation of this is awaited.

Rheumatoid arthritis

Rheumatoid arthritis is the commonest chronic inflammatory joint disease. It may, however, affect any organ within the body, including the eye. The commonest ocular problem seen in RA is secondary SS occurring in 25% of patients (see Sjögren's syndrome). Scleritis and particularly scleromalacia perforans may have devastating effects on the eye and result in a profound loss of vision.

Aetiology

The prevalence of rheumatoid arthritis (RA) is approximately 3% and whilst this has been increasing during this century it would now appear to have peaked. There is a female:male ratio of 3:1. A strong genetic predisposition for RA is evident. For example, 60% of those with RA are HLA DR4 positive compared with a prevalence of 30% in the general population[22]. The initial trigger for RA remains unknown although various studies have implicated a number of organisms. The role of dietary and psychological factors remains unclear.

The immunopathology of rheumatoid arthritis

Whilst rheumatoid arthritis is clearly a disease that focuses on the synovial tissues, it is also a multisystemic disease — the heart, lungs, central nervous system and skin may all be involved. As with the other autoimmune diseases, a wide variety of defects have been found in most of the cellular compartments of the immune system. Recent intense research efforts have focused on the MHC Class II expression of synovial cells and the role of cytokines. Thus, rheumatoid inflammatory synovial cells seem to have the same characteristics as lymphoid dendritic cells. For example, the synovial cells are positive for Class II MHC antigens and the common leukocyte

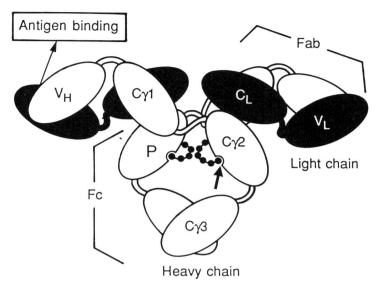

Figure 9.3 The site of inter-linked oligosaccharides is seen in the Cγ2 domain. Absence of the terminal sialic acid and galactose residues (see text) might 'empty' the pocket (arrowed) into which they normally bind, or expose amino acid sequences usually concealed by the oligosaccharide chains

antigen, but lack other mononuclear cell markers. Rheumatoid dendritic cells produce significant quantities of IL-1, which is thought to be capable of triggering T cells and maturing B cells and also to be involved in synovial tissue destruction[23].

Serologically, the most striking abnormality is the presence of auto-antibodies directed against the Fc region of the body's own IgG. In the last two years, major attempts have been made to elucidate this, by an analysis of the carbohydrate moieties that bridge the Cγ2 domain. In particular, it has been shown that the bi-antennary arms of the oligosaccharide chains that are attached to each Cγ2 region are deficient in the terminal sialic acid and galactose sugars[24]. Under normal circumstances, the interaction of these two chains is responsible both for maintaining the structure of this part of the Fc region, and also for concealing certain amino acids found in this area (Figure 9.3). Although the lack of terminal galactose studies is in part an age-related phenomenon[25], extensive studies have shown that patients with rheumatoid arthritis have a very high percentage of IgG molecules that are relatively agalactosylated[26]. This could render the Cγ2 domain immunogenic by a variety of pathways, notably by exposing amino acids that are not normally seen by the immune system, or by the lectin-like activity of the truncated oligosaccharide arms.

High levels of immune complexes can be found in synovial fluid, and the evidence suggests that the joint is indeed the site of their formation. Joint damage probably occurs owing to the inflammatory effect of complement-

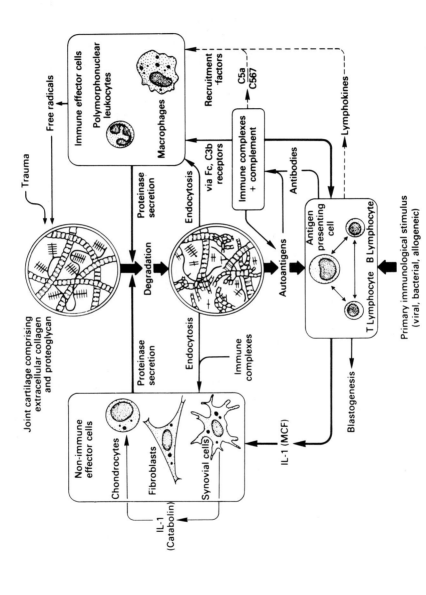

Figure 9.4 Guide to the immunopathology of rheumatoid arthritis. The cycle is probably triggered by infection, although it is conceivable that trauma alone might trigger the inflammatory cascade. After the primary event, in a suitably predisposed host, a series of steps occur that lead to autosensitization against cartilage components, inflammation and joint damage.

fixing immune complexes that can recruit polymorphonuclear leukocytes into the joint, where they may release lysozymal enzymes[4]. Free radicals may also be generated by the respiratory burst from these neutrophils, and they too could contribute to further tissue damage. A suggested cycle of events is shown in Figure 9.4.

Juvenile chronic arthritis

Chronic arthritis presenting under the age of 16 years is termed juvenile chronic arthritis (JCA) in Europe and juvenile rheumatoid arthritis (JRA) in North America. JCA encompasses a number of clinically distinct groups. Three of these are at risk of developing ocular complications: pauciarticular JCA, polyarticular JCA and juvenile ankylosing spondylitis (see "juvenile ankylosing spondylitis" below).

Pauciarticular JCA

The diagnosis of pauciarticular JCA is made on the basis of persistent arthritis affecting three or fewer joints for longer than 3 months. Patients are seronegative for RhF. Chronic anterior uveitis occurs in 63–91% of cases. A particular subset who are female and less than 5 years old at age of disease onset with a positive ANA have been shown to be at increased risk of developing chronic anterior uveitis[27,28]. However, whether the ANAs detected in these patients are simply a marker of disease or involved in its immuno-pathology remains uncertain. The clinical importance of this is that most patients are asymptomatic in the initial stages of developing uveitis, but progression of the disease is a cause of major morbidity[29,30]. It may present in a minority with the insidious onset of blurred vision, loss of visual acuity or ocular pain.

Ocular findings may include the presence of a flare in the anterior chamber, keratitic precipitates (KPs), posterior synechiae, band keratopathy (34%), cataract (39%), glaucoma (20%), phthisis (5%) and rarely posterior uveitis (<3%)[31].

The disease activities of the arthritis and uveitis usually run an independent course[32]. An early onset of uveitis in relation to arthritis appears to be associated with a poor prognosis. There is evidence in children with juvenile chronic arthritis and uveitis of immunity to ocular antigen, although a pathogenic role is not proven[31].

Polyarticular JCA

This group with seronegative polyarticular disease overlaps considerably with pauciarticular JCA: 12–37% are at risk of developing chronic anterior uveitis[31].

Scleroderma

Scleroderma is a generalized disorder of connective tissue resulting in diffuse fibrosis of the dermis. Subdermal tissues and internal organs, particularly the gastrointestinal tract, lung, kidneys and heart may also be affected.

The only ocular problem associated with scleroderma is secondary Sjögren's syndrome, occurring in 17% of patients[1].

The immunopathology of scleroderma

The pathogenesis of scleroderma has at least three elements: the vascular abnormalities, the immunological perturbations, and the disordered collagen synthesis. It seems very likely that the primary vascular event found in the small blood vessels is the proliferation of endothelial cells in the intimal layer[33]. Disruption of the endothelial lining cells occurs and this is followed by a proliferation of smooth muscle cells and associated with damage of the blood vessel wall. It is reasonable to propose that the endothelial cell damage may occur in reponse to ischaemia[34], of which Raynaud's phenomenon may simply be the most obvious manifestation.

It is, however, the greatly accelerated rate of fibroblast collagen synthesis that is the key to the immunopathology of this disease. Whether it is the lack of control mechanisms that limits the amount of collagen made by fibroblasts or that there is indeed something abnormal about the fibroblasts themselves remains the subject of much speculation. There is certainly evidence of increased release and activity of IL-1[35].

Like most autoimmune diseases, scleroderma is more common among women and has also been linked to HLA antigens B8, DR3 and DR5. Serologically, the disease is characterized by the presence of antinuclear antibodies that are present in over 90% of these patients. At least two antibodies, those binding the centromere (30–40%) and anti-Scl-70 antibodies (25%), appear to be disease-specific. The Scl-70 antigen has been identified as an enzyme topoisomerase 1[36]. This enzyme unwinds the helical form of single-stranded DNA in preparation for gene replication. It has recently been suggested that a selective vulnerability to the action of topoisomerase 1 is built into the structure of dermal collagen genes[37].

Early in the disease, cellular infiltrates composed of lymphocytes, plasma cells and macrophages are commonly found, especially as a perivascular cuff of skin biopsies[4]. Analyses of skin sections have shown that the majority of these cells are T-lymphocytes, and other evidence exists that supports the potential role of cell-mediated immune mechanisms in the aetiopathogenesis of scleroderma. A proposed pathway of events is shown in Figure 9.5.

SERONEGATIVE SPONDARTHRITIDES

The group of diseases designated seronegative spondarthritides share certain common distinctive features suggesting a linked pathogenesis. Amongst these features, the frequent finding of HLA-B27 is notable. The group includes ankylosing spondylitis (AS), Reiter's syndrome, arthropathy associated with inflammatory bowel disease and psoriatic arthropathy.

The clinical characteristics include radiological sacroiliitis, an asymmetrical lower-limb large-joint arthropathy, negative RhF, a familial tendency and

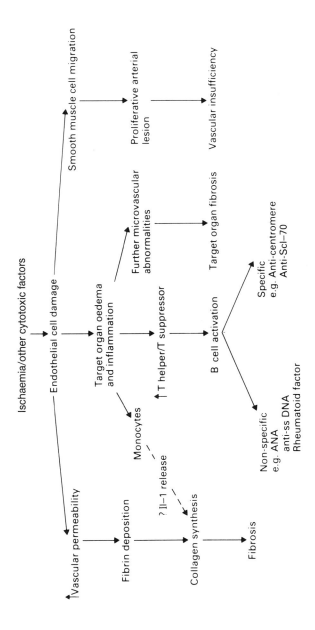

Figure 9.5 Suggested complex interactions including vascular, endothelial and immunological factors associated with the immunopathology of scleroderma. (Reproduced with permission from Morrow, W. J. W. and Isenberg, D. A. *Autoimmune Rheumatic Disease.* (Oxford: Blackwell Scientific))

overlapping extra-articular features. These last include uveitis and conjunctivitis, cardiovascular disease, e.g. aortic incompetence, pericarditis and conduction defects and upper lobe pulmonary fibrosis.

The hallmark of eye disease in seronegative arthritis is anterior uveitis.

Ankylosing spondylitis

Conjunctivitis and uveitis may occur in up to 25% of patients during their illness. Uveitis may be a presenting feature in 10% of patients with AS[38]. The diagnosis of AS should therefore be considered in any young male with recurrent anterior uveitis. Uveitis is associated with peripheral joint involvement but not the severity of spondylitis[39].

The immunopathology of ankylosing spondylitis

This condition has an incidence approaching 1–2%, with a male:female ratio of 3:1. It has an extremely strong association with HLA B27, which is present in 96% of cases. The prevalence of HLA B27 in the general population is 4–8%. However, the disease occurs in only 1% of carriers with HLA B27. An environmental trigger is therefore involved and Gram-negative bacteria have been implicated. In particular, there is evidence of cross-reactivity between klebsiella cell wall components and the HLA B27 molecule[40]. The presence of klebsiella in the stool is associated with activation of uveitis but not AS activity[41].

Juvenile ankylosing spondylitis

This group of patients consists principally of boys over 10 years of age, with sacroiliitis, spinal involvement and large-joint arthropathy. Reactive arthritis and arthropathy associated with inflammatory bowel disease may also occur in children, with similar features to those of adult onset disease. There is a strong association with HLA B27. They may suffer with acute recurrent anterior uveitis in up to 25% of cases[42].

Reiter's syndrome

The classic triad of Reiter's syndrome involves a precipitating infection, either a non-specific urethritis or bacillary dysentery along with an asymmetrical reactive arthritis and inflammatory eye disease, commonly anterior uveitis or conjunctivitis.

Anterior uveitis occurs in the acute syndrome some 4–6 weeks after the primary trigger. Symptoms are frequently mild. Uveitis, which may be very severe, occurs in up to 30% of cases with chronic disease especially if sacroiliitis is present.

Reiter's syndrome has been found to include keratoderma blennorrhagia, circinate balanitis, sacroiliitis, enthesopathy and tendonitis. The natural history may be short-lived but a proportion of patients suffer chronic or recurrent disease[43].

The immunopathology of Reiter's syndrome

The disease predominantly affects young males and is associated with HLA B27. Precipitating factors include chlamydia as a cause of non-specific urethritis (NSU) and shigella, salmonella and yersinia causing dysentery. The pathogenic mechanisms of the reactive arthritis and uveitis are unclear. Chlamydia have been isolated from synovial fluid[44-46] and chlamydial antigen has been isolated from synovial biopsies[47-49]. Cross-reactivity between chlamydial antigen and HLA B27 may explain host damage[50]. Vascular changes similar to those produced by circulating endotoxins have been demonstrated[51] and immunoglobulin has been shown to be present around vessel walls in reactive arthritis[52].

A number of animal models exist that show some of the characteristics seen in ocular disease associated with immune disorders. For example, injection of strains of mycoplasma arthritidis into experimental animals produces a chronic synovitis and an acute uveitis similar to that seen in Reiter's syndrome and related seronegative spondarthritides[53].

SYSTEMIC VASCULITIDES

Polyarteritis nodosa

Polyarteritis nodosa (PAN) is a rare necrotizing vasculitis of small and medium-sized arteries.

Eye involvement occurs in 40–80% of patients. This may be scleritis or less commonly anterior uveitis. The choroidal and retinal circulations show evidence of vasculitis and in the retina, haemorrhages and cotton-wool spots are seen in 10–20% of cases. Central retinal artery occlusion, ischaemic optic neuropathy and macular oedema may also result in profound visual loss. A rare complication is granulomatous involvement of the orbit, resulting in proptosis, diplopia and loss of vision.

Multisystem involvement may result in glomerulonephritis, acute renal failure, hypertension, mononeuritis multiplex, cutaneous ulcers, intestinal infarction and perforation.

The immunopathology of PAN

Histological findings are non-specific, showing focal inflammatory cell infiltration, necrosis and fibrosis of affected vessels.

The basic immunopathological process may well be immune-complex-mediated. Animal studies, notably the acute serum sickness model in rabbits, confirm that immune-complex formation may be associated with necrotizing arteritis[54]. This model is closely mirrored in PAN, where there are initially endothelial changes and immune-complex deposition, subsequently inflammatory infiltration predominantly with polymorphonuclear cells, and finally chronic inflammation leading to scarring. The antigenic component of the immune complexes remains unidentified. The association between hepatitis B and PAN first reported at about 30%, is now recognized to be much lower at

6–8%. Circulating immune complexes containing HBSAg have been demonstrated in PAN but are also described in chronic active hepatitis without vasculitis. It is thus improbable that persistent carriage of HBSAg has a significant role in the aetiology of PAN.

Giant-cell arteritis

Giant-cell arteritis consists of a spectrum of disease from the relatively mild polymyalgia rheumatica to the potentially life-threatening cranial arteritis. It is a large-vessel vasculitis affecting the cranial branches of arteries arising from the aortic arch. Visual features are a presenting complaint in 6% of cases. Ocular symptoms include amaurosis fugax, blurred vision, diplopia, transient and permanent blindness. Most of these symptoms are related to ischaemic changes affecting the optic nerve and less commonly the central retinal artery.

The condition is rare under the age of 50 years with a mean age of onset of 65–75 years. The majority of patients are female. Typically, the presentation is with temporal headaches and tenderness, associated with malaise, fever and stiffness, particularly affecting the upper limbs.

Findings on examination include the presence of tender, thickened temporal arteries. There may in addition be a synovitis of peripheral joints similar to that seen in RA. Proximal muscles are often tender but weakness is not a feature.

Laboratory findings include a normochromic normocytic anaemia and a high erythrocyte sedimentation rate (ESR). This may be greater than 100 mm/h but a result greater than 40 mm/h is good evidence of activity. A small proportion of patients have a normal ESR, in which case the C-reactive protein (CRP) is often raised. Temporal artery biopsy may demonstrate arteritis including the presence of vessel narrowing, fibrinoid necrosis, destruction of the internal elastic lamina and giant cells.

The immunopathology of GCA

Circumstantial evidence supports an underlying immunological abnormality in GCA. Elevated serum IgG and complement levels are commonly found. Immunoglobulin and complement deposition in temporal artery biopsies has been demonstrated. It is unclear whether these complexes derive from circulating immune complexes or whether antibodies bind to antigen *in situ*. In addition, immunohistological evidence of large numbers of T cells, predominantly T-helper CD4+ cells, has been demonstrated[55]. The relative importance of immune-complex and cell-mediated damage remains unclear.

A genetic predisposition is possible, with a significant increase in HLA DR3 and DR4 demonstrated in one study[56]. The disease is much more common in caucasians and familial aggregation has also been described.

Behçet's disease

Behçet's disease is a multisystem vasculitic disease. Ocular involvement results in recurrent bilateral non-granulomatous uveitis in 75% of patients. This may be anterior, posterior or a panuveitis. Conjunctivitis, scleritis and keratitis may also occur. Posterior uveitis is often severe and can result in macular oedema, causing visual loss. Both arterial and venous sheathing and occlusions may occur. Neovascularization, often causing vitreous haemorrage, may occur in ischaemic areas.

The triad of recurrent oral and genital ulceration and uveitis should be widened to include multisystem involvement of skin, joints, venous thrombosis, gastrointestinal, cardiovascular and central nervous systems.

The immunopathology of Behçet's disease

There is a strong association with HLAB5/B51 subtype in some ethnic groups, suggesting a genetic predisposition[57]. The search for a putative infective organism has been exhaustive and there is a tenuous relationship with streptococcal organisms. The possibility that this is a viral disease was postulated by Behçet himself and virus-like particles in vitreous fluid have been described[58]. Evidence suggesting immune-complex-mediated damage, particularly for eye and joint complications, includes the demonstration of circulating immune complexes and deposition of immunoglobulin and complement in tissue from patients with Behçet's. More recently, evidence for the possible role of herpes simplex type 1 virus (HSV-1) has accumulated. HSV-1 specific IgG1 circulating immune complexes have been described. Excess copies of HSV-RNA and DNA have been demonstrated in lymphocytes of some patients with Behçet's. A decreased proliferative response of CD4+ cells when stimulated by HSV-1 was also demonstrated in comparison to controls[59]. Conversely, there is an excessive response by CD8+ (suppressor) T cells. This suggests a T-cell defect in immunoregulation following viral infection.

Antibodies to mucosal cells have been demonstrated in Behçet's but these are non-specific and are also found in aphthous ulceration[60].

Wegener's granulomatosis

Wegener's granulomatosis is a necrotizing granulomatous vasculitis affecting upper and lower respiratory tracts, often combined with a glomerulonephritis. A limited form is recognized in the absence of renal involvement. Ocular features may be seen in over 40% of subjects. The primary clinical problem may be a vasculitis affecting the eye. Ocular findings include scleritis, uveitis, optic nerve vasculitis, cotton-wool spots, choroidal and retinal detachment, and retinal arteritis[61,62]. Rarely, there may be granulomatous involvement of the orbit.

The immunopathology of Wegner's granulomatosis

The principal pathological features include necrotizing granulomata of the respiratory tract and focal segmental necrotizing glomerulonephritis. Crescent formation is common. Both circulating and deposited immune complexes have been demonstrated in a proportion of cases, but the significance remains unclear. There is a notable lack of immune-complex deposition in renal biopsies of patients with glomerulonephritis[63].

An immune aetiology is supported by the finding of antineutrophil cytoplasmic antibody in 90% of patients with Wegener's. The antibodies are not disease-specific, being found in a number of other forms of systemic vasculitis. It is proposed that they are formed as a fundamental part of the process of systemic vasculitis and not merely as a result of endothelial cell damage, since they are absent in Henoch–Schönlein disease. Antibody titre appears to be related to disease activity. Evidence suggests that the autoantigen for these antibodies is associated with alkaline phosphatase[64], though this is now disputed.

Sarcoidosis

Sarcoidosis is a systemic granulomatous disorder. The clinical presentation is usually divided into acute and chronic forms. The commonly affected organ systems include skin (erythema nodosum, lupus pernio), lung (pulmonary fibrosis), reticuloendothelial system (lymphadenopathy, hepatosplenomegaly), nervous system (peripheral neuropathy, mononeuritis multiplex) and musculoskeletal (arthritis, tenosynovitis). Ocular involvement occurs in 25% of cases. There may be a non-specific conjunctivitis or involvement of the eyelids and conjunctiva with granulomata. Lacrimal gland enlargement and infiltration may lead to keratoconjunctivitis sicca. The most common feature is uveitis. In the acute presentation this is usually acute anterior uveitis with erythema nodosum and hilar lymphadenopathy. Chronic anterior uveitis may be associated with lupus pernio and pulmonary fibrosis. Posterior uveal involvement may occur together with retinal vasculitis, macular oedema and optic neuropathy, all of which can cause visual loss.

The immunopathology of sarcoidosis

A disordered immune system in sarcoidosis is clear from the common clinical findings of hypergammaglobulinaemia and a negative tuberculin test (in patients who have had BCG vaccination or tuberculosis in the past), indicating apparent impaired cellular immunity. There is peripheral lymphopenia and reduced CD4+ and B-cell function.

The initiating agent remains unclear but possibly acts on the lungs, where pulmonary alveolar macrophages are activated, expressing IL-2 receptors[65], and through antigen presentation and lymphokine production (IL-1 and INF-γ) promote proliferation and activation of lymphocytes and fibroblasts, resulting in granuloma formation and fibrosis[66]. In marked contrast to the case in peripheral blood, T-cell numbers in the lungs are increased, principally CD4+ cells, showing activation markers[67]. The pathology of sarcoidosis is thus explained, at least in part, by sequestration and activation of the immune system at focal sites particularly the lungs.

Relapsing polychondritis

Relapsing polychondritis is a rare systemic disorder of unknown aetiology affecting cartilage. Ocular features include conjunctivitis, keratitis, scleritis and uveitis. Persistent inflammation results in destruction of the pinna of the ear, nasal septum and upper airways. Associated features include a non-erosive arthritis. Thirty per cent have an associated autoimmune disease. Death commonly ensues if airway obstruction and pneumonia develop. The 5-year mortality rate is 25%.

The immunopathology of relapsing polychondritis

There is some evidence of immune pathology in relapsing polychondritis (RPC). Antibodies directed against cartilage matrix and type II collagen have been described. They appear to be present early in the disease course, suggesting pathogenicity[68]. Enchanced cell-mediated immunity against cartilage proteoglycans has also been described[69]. In addition, RPC has been associated with other autoimmune disorders including rheumatoid arthritis, systemic lupus erythematosus, Sjögren's syndrome and recently in a patient with myasthenia gravis and thymoma[70].

ORGAN-SPECIFIC DISEASES

Graves's disease

Autoimmune thyroid eye disease, or Graves's disease, is the commonest cause of unilateral or bilateral proptosis. Other ocular features include proptosis, lid lag and retraction, chemosis, superior limbic keratitis and, rarely, optic nerve compression. The latter may result in decreased visual acuity, a central-field defect and an afferent pupillary defect.

The immunopathology of Graves's disease

The close relationship of Graves's ophthalmopathy (GO) to autoimmune thyroid disease strongly supports an autoimmune aetiology. Histological studies in early GO show interstitial oedema and cellular infiltration of external ocular muscles. Principal cell types are lymphocytes, plasma cells and macrophages. The lesion progresses to fibrosis and muscle-fibre atrophy.

At present, there is no evidence to suggest that the numerous antibodies directed against thyroid tissue (LATS, TSI, TSII thyroid microsomal antibody) and TSH itself cause ophthalmopathy

Evidence of specific cell-mediated immunity to external ocular antigen has been reported, suggesting the existence of different subsets of T cells in the pathogenesis of GO and thyroid disease. A defect in specific suppressor T-cell subsets is proposed. However, attempts to reproduce some of these data have failed[71].

Aberrant expression of Class II antigens on thyroid cells that might then act as additional antigen-presenting cells of autoantigens may be important in perpetuating autoimmune thyroid disease[72].

Antibodies to external ocular muscle antigens have been described, but their specificity remains in doubt because of the crude nature of the antigen preparations used. It is also unclear whether these antibodies are pathogenic or arise secondary to the tissue damage.

Myasthenia gravis

Myasthenia gravis is an uncommon disorder of neuromuscular transmission. The commonest presentation involves external ocular, bulbar, neck and shoulder girdle muscles. Ocular findings include ptosis, diplopia and occasionally complete ophthalmoplegia. The weakness is characteristically fatiguable. The diagnosis is based on the clinical picture, electromyographic studies showing fatiguability with supramaximal stimulation, a positive response to edrophonium (Tensilon test) and the presence of AChR antibody.

The immunopathology of myasthenia gravis

There is overwhelming evidence that myasthenia gravis (MG) is an autoimmune disorder. Immunoglobulin has been demonstrated at the neuromuscular end-plate. When purified, this shows acetylcholine receptor (AChR) binding. Transfer of these antibodies to mice induces neuromuscular blockade. Similarly, infants born to mothers with MG show transient myasthenia until maternal IgG is cleared.

Serum complement levels are reduced; C3 and C9 have been demonstrated on the postsynaptic membrane. Antibody-dependent complement-mediated damage to the postsynaptic membrane is a proposed mechanism because *in vitro* fixing of complement by anti-AChR antibody (AChR Ab) occurs. Other effects include blocking of AChR by antibody but this is partial and so probably plays only a minor role[73]. In addition, enhanced turnover of AChR induced by AChR Ab has been demonstrated.

The role of the thymus remains unclear. It has been demonstrated to be an unusual site of germinal-centre formation and thus of B-cell production in MG. AChR is expressed on myoid and epithelial cells present in the thymus. Thymus-derived B cells show enhanced activation and immunoglobulin production compared to controls. Although this may in part be polyclonal, there is some evidence that they produce more AChR Ab than peripheral cells. The thymus might therefore be an important site for the initiation or perpetuation of the immune response in MG.

Antibodies directed against epitopes on other antibodies (anti-idiotypes) play an important role in immune regulation. The demonstration of anti-idiotypes in MG raises the possibility that whilst these may in part be protective they may also be harmful, by stimulating autoantibody synthesis[74].

CONCLUSION

It is clear that ocular involvement is an important manifestation of disease in both the 'classical' autoimmune disorders and related rheumatological conditions. We have reviewed the current state of knowledge of the immunopathogenesis of these conditions. Some conditions have a clear immune basis, whilst in others the relationship is less obvious. It is very likely that both cellular and humoral mechanisms are involved in an integrated way in the immunopathology of most of the diseases we have discussed. Future work unravelling the complexities of the immunopathology will enable us to gain a clearer understanding of these diseases and perhaps point to new avenues of treatment.

References

1. Maddison, P. J. (1985). Dry eyes: Autoimmunity and relationship to other systemic disease. *Trans. Ophthalmol. Soc. U.K.*, **104**, 458–61
2. Strand, V. and Talal, N. (1980). Advances in the diagnosis and concept of Sjögren's syndrome (autoimmune endocrinopathy). *Bull. Rheum. Dis.*, **14**, 77–105
3. Fox, R. I., Howell, F. V., Bone, R. L. *et al.* (1984). Primary Sjögren's syndrome: clinical and immunopathological features. *Semin. Arthritis Rheum.*, **14**, 77–105
4. Morrow, W. J. W. and Isenberg, D. A. (1987). *Autoimmune Rheumatic Disease*. (Oxford: Blackwell Scientific)
5. Horsfall, A. C., Venables, P. J. W., Allard, S. A. and Maini, R. N. (1988). Co-existent anti-La antibodies and rheumatoid factors bear distinct idiotypic markers. *Scand. J. Rheumatol.*, **Suppl. 75**, 84–8
6. Venables, P. (1988). Sjögren's syndrome: differential diagnosis, immunopathology and genetics. In Scott, T., Dieppe, P., Moll, J. and Isenberg, D. A. (eds.) *Topical Reviews, Reports on Rheumatic Diseases*, p. 10. (London: ARC Publications)
7. Coles, R. S. (1985). Ocular manifestations of connective tissue disease. *Hosp. Pract.*, **20** (2), 70–6
8. Dubois, E. L. (1974). The clinical picture of systemic lupus erythematosus. In Dubois, E. L. (ed.) *Lupus Erythematosus*, pp. 323–6. (Los Angeles: University of Southern California Press)
9. Bishko, F. (1972). Retinopathy in systemic lupus erythematosus: a case report and review of the literature. *Arthritis Rheum.*, **15**, 57–63
10. Lanham, I. G., Barrie, T., Kolmer, E. M. and Hughes, G. R. V. (1982). SLE retinopathy: evaluation by fluorescein angiography. *Ann. Rheum. Dis.*, **41**, 473–8
11. Coppeto, J. and Lessel, S. (1977). Retinopathy in systemic lupus erythematosus. *Arch. Ophthalmol.*, **95**, 794–7
12. Lachman, S. and Hazleman, B. (1975). Rheumatic diseases and the eye. *Hosp. Update*, (Oct), 613–33
13. Stafford-Brady, F. J., Urowitz, M. B., Gladman, D. D. and Easterbrook, M. (1988). Lupus retinopathy: patterns, associations and prognosis. *Arthritis Rheum.*, **31** (9), 1105–10
14. Fessel, W. J. (1974). Systemic lupus erythematosus in the community. *Arch. Intern. Med.*, **134**, 1027
15. Nobrega, F. T., Fergusson, R. H., Kurland, L. T. *et al.* (1968). Lupus erythematosus Rochester, Minnesota, 1950–1965. A preliminary study. In Bennett, P. H. and Wood, P. H. N. (eds.) *Population Studies of the Rheumatic Diseases*, p. 259. Proceedings of the Third International Congress, Series 148 (New York: Excerpta Medica Foundation)
16. Block, S. R., Winfield, J. B., Lockshin, M. *et al.* (1975). Studies of twins with systemic lupus erythematosus. A review of the literature and presentation of 12 additional sets. *Am. J. Med.*, **59**, 193
17. Dar, O., Salaman, M. R., Seifert, M. H. and Isenberg, D. A. (1988). B-lymphocyte activation in systemic lupus erythematosus: spontaneous production of IgG antibodies to DNA and environmental antigens in cultures of blood mononuclear cells. *Clin. Exp. Immunol.*, **73**, 430–5
18. Lebon, P., Lenoir, G. R., Fischer, A. and Lagrue, A. (1984). Synthesis of intrathecal interferon in systemic lupus erythematosus with neurological complications. *Br. Med. J.*, **287**, 1105–7
19. Shoenfeld, Y. and Isenberg, D. A. (1987). DNA antibody idiotypes: A review of their genetic, clinical and immunopathological features. *Semin. Arthritis Rheum.*, **16**, 245–52

20. Chen, P. P., Liv, M. R., Sinha, S. and Carson, D. A. (1988). A 16/6 idiotype positive anti-DNA antibody is encoded by a conserved V_H gene with no somatic mutation. *Arthritis Rheum.*, **31**, 1429–31
21. Mendelovic, S., Brocker, S., Shoenfeld, Y. *et al.*, (1988). Induction of a systemic lupus erythematosus-like disease in mice by a common human anti-DNA idiotype. *Proc. Natl. Acad. Sci. USA*, **85**, 2260–4
22. Strastny, P. (1978). Association of the B-cell alloantigen DRW4 with rheumatoid arthritis. *N. Engl. J. Med.*, **298**, 869
23. Waaler, K., Forre, O. and Natvig, J. B. (1988). Dendritic cells in rheumatoid inflammation. *Springer Semin Inmmunopathol.*, **10**, 141–56
24. Parekh, R. B., Dwek, R. A., Sutton, B. *et al.* (1985). Association of rheumatoid arthritis and primary osteoarthritis with changes in the glycosylation pattern of total serum IgG. *Nature*, **316**, 452–6
25. Parekh, R. B., Isenberg, D. A., Roitt, I. M., Dwek, R. A. and Rademacher, T. W. (1988). Age-related galactosylation of the N-linked oligosaccharides of human serum IgG. *J. Exp. Med.*, **167**, 1731–6
26. Rademacher, T. W., Parekh, R. B., Dwek, R. A. *et al.* (1988). The role of IgG glycoforms in the pathogenesis of rheumatoid arthritis. *Springer Semin. Immunopathol.*, **10**, 231–50
27. Petty, R. E., Cassidy, J. T. and Sullivan, D. B. (1973). Clinical correlates of antinuclear antibodies in juvenile rheumatoid arthritis. *J. Pediatr.*, **83**, 386–9
28. Kanshii, J. J. and Shum-Shin, G. A. (1984). Systemic uveitis syndromes: an analysis of 340 cases. *Ophthalmology*, **91**, 1240–52
29. Schaller, J., Smiley, W. K. and Ansell, B. M. (1973). Iridocyclitis of juvenile rheumatoid arthritis (JRA Still's disease). *Arthritis Rheum.*, **16**, 130–1 (abst.)
30. Schaller, R. G., Johnson, G. D., Holborrow, E. J. *et al.* (1974). The association of antinuclear antibodies with chronic iridocyclitis of juvenile rheumatoid arthritis (Still's disease). *Arthritis Rheum.*, **17**, 409–16
31. Petty, R. E. (1987). Current knowledge of the etiology and pathogenesis of chronic uveitis accompanying juvenile rheumatoid arthritis. *Rheum. Dis. Clin. N. Am.*, **16**, 19–36
32. Rosenberg, A. M. (1987). Uveitis associated with juvenile rheumatoid arthritis. *Semin. Arthritis Rheum.*, **16** (3), 158–73
33. Fleischmajer, R. and Perlish, J. S. (1980). Capillary alterations in scleroderma. *J. Am. Acad. Dermatol.*, **2**, 161–70
34. Lee, E. B., Anhalt, G. J., Voorkees, J. J. and Diaz, L. A. (1984). Pathogenesis of scleroderma. Current concepts. *Int. J. Dermatol.*, **22**, 85–9
35. Whiteside, T. L., Worrall, J. G., Prince, R. K., Buckingham, R. B. and Rodnan, G. P. (1985). Soluble mediators from mononuclear cells increase the synthesis of glycosamino-glycan by dermal fibroblast cultures derived from normal subjects and progressive systemic sclerosis patients. *Arthritis Rheum.*, **28**, 188–97
36. Sheva, J. H., Bardwell, B., Rothfield, N. F. and Earnshaw, W. C. (1986). High titres of autoantibodies to topoisomerase I, (Scl-70) in sera from scleroderma patients. *Science*, **231**, 737–40
37. Douvas, A. (1988). Does Scl-70 modulate collagen production in systemic sclerosis? *Lancet*, **2**, 475–7
38. Wilkinson, M. and Bywaters, E. (1958). Clinical features and course of ankylosing spondylitis as seen in a follow-up of 22 hospital referral cases. *Ann. Rheum. Dis.*, **17**, 209
39. Lehtien, K. (1983). 76 patients with anklosing spondylitis seen after 30 years of disease. *Scand. J. Rheumatol.*, **12**, 5–11
40. Ebringer, A. (1983). The cross-tolerance hypothesis. HLA-B27 and ankylosing spondylitis. *Br. J. Rheumatol.*, **22**, (suppl. 2), 53–66
41. Ebringer, R., Cooke, D., Cowdell, D. R. *et al.* (1977). Ankylosing spondylitis klebsiella and HLA B27. *Rheumatol. Rehab.*, **16**, 190–6
42. Allen, R. C. and Ansell, B. M. (1986). Juvenile chronic arthritis — clinical sub-groups with particular relationship to adult patterns of disease. *Postgrad. Med. J.*, **62**, 821–6
43. Calin, A. (1984). Reiter's syndrome. In Calin, A. (ed.) *Spondyloarthropathies*, pp. 119–49. (Orlando: Grune and Stratton)
44. Dunlop, E. M. C., Harper, I. A. and Jones, B. R. (1968). Seronegative polyarthritis: the Bedsonia (Chlamydia) group of agents and Reiter's disease. *Ann. Rheum. Dis.*, **27**, 234–40

45. Engleman, E. P., Schacter, J., Gilbert, R. J. *et al.* (1969). Bedsonia and Reiter's syndrome: a progress report. *Arthritis Rheum.*, **12**, 292 (abst.)
46. Vilppula, A. H., Yli-Kertlula, V. L., Ahloos, A. K. *et al.* (1981). Chlamydial isolation and serology in Reiter's syndrome. *Scand J. Rheumatol.*, **10**, 181–5
47. Schumacher, H. R., Cherian, P. V., Sieck, M. *et al.* (1986). Ultrastructural identification of chlamydial antigens in synovial membrane in acute Reiter's syndrome. 50th American Rheumatism Association Meeting, New Orleans. *Arthritis Rheum.*, **29** (Suppl): Abstract 115
48. Kent, A., Thomas, B., Dixey, J. *et al.* (1987). Chlamydia trachomatis and reactive arthritis — The missing link. *Lancet*, **1**, 72–4
49. Schumacher, H. R., Magge, S., Cherian, V. *et al.* (1988). Light and electron microscopic studies on the synovial membrane in Reiter's syndrome. Immunocytochemical idenfication of chlamydial antigen in patients with early disease. *Arthritis Rheum.*, **31**, 937–46
50. Inman, R. D. (1986). The interplay of microbe and MHC in the pathogenesis of Reiter's syndrome. *Clin. Exp. Rheumatol.*, **4**, 75–82
51. Norton, W. L., Lewis, D. and Ziff, M. (1966). Light and electron microscopic observations on the synovitis of Reiter's syndrome. *Arthritis Rheum.*, **9**, 947–57
52. Balassare, A. R., Weiss, T. D., Tsai, C. C. *et al.* (1981). Immunoprotein deposition in synovial tissue in Reiter's syndrome. *Ann. Rheum. Dis.*, **40**, 281–5
53. Thurkill, C. E. and Gregson, D. S. (1982). Mycoplasma arthritidis-induced ocular inflammatory disease. *Infect. Immun.*, **36**, 775–81
54. Editorial (1985). Systemic vasculitis. *Lancet*, **1**, 1252
55. Banks, P. M., Cohen, D., Ginsburg, W. W. and Hunder, G. G. (1983). Immunohistologic and cytochemical studies of temporal arteritis. *Arthritis Rheum.*, **26**, 1201–7
56. Lowenstein, M. B., Bridgeford, P. H., Vasey, F. *et al.* (1983). Increased frequency of HLA-DR3 and DR4 in polymyalgia rheumatica — giant cell arteritis. *Arthritis Rheum.*, **26**, 925–7
57. Ohno, S., Asamima, T., Suiguira, S. *et al.* (1978). HLA BW51 and Behçet's disease. *J. Am. Med. Assoc.*, **240**, 259
58. Sezer, F. N. (1956). The isolation of a virus as the cause of Behçet's disease. *Am. J. Ophthalmol.*, **41**, 41
59. Lehner, T. (1986). The role of a disorder in immunoregulation associated with Herpes simplex type I in Behçet's disease. In Lehner, T. and Barnes, C. G. (eds.). *Recent Advances in Behçet's Disease*, pp. 31–36. RSM International Congress and Symposium Series No. 103. (London: Royal Society of Medicine)
60. Oshima, Y., Shimizu, T., Yokohari, R. *et al.* (1963). Clinical studies on Behçet's syndrome. *Ann. Rheum. Dis.*, **22**, 36
61. Haynes, B. F., Fishman, M. L., Fauci, A. S. *et al.* (1977). The ocular manifestations of Wegener's granulomatosus: Fifteen years experience and review of the literature. *Am. J. Med.*, **63**, 131–41
62. Leveille, A. S. and Morse, P. H. (1981). Combined detachments in Wegener's granulomatosus. *Br. J. Ophthalmol.*, **65**, 564–7
63. Cupps, T. R. and Fauci, A. S. (1981). *The Vasculitides* (Philadelphia: W. B. Saunders)
64. Lockwood, C. M., Bankes, D., Jones, S. *et al.* (1987). Association of alkaline phosphatase with an autoantigen recognized by circulating anti-neutrophil antibodies in systemic vasculitis. *Lancet*, **1**, 716–20
65. Hanock, W. W., Kobzik, L. and Colby, A. J. (1986). Detection of lymphokines and lymphokine receptors in pulmonary sarcoidosis. *Am. J. Pathol.*, **123**, 1–8
66. Venet, A., Hance, A., Saltini, C. *et al.* (1985). Enhanced alveolar macrophage mediated antigen-induced T lymphocyte proliferation in sarcoidosis. *J. Clin. Invest.*, **75**, 293–301
67. Pinkston, P., Bitterman, P. B. and Crystal, R. G. (1983). Spontaneous release of interleukin-2 by T lymphocytes in active pulmonary sarcoidosis. *N. Engl. J. Med.*, **308**, 793–800
68. Ebringer, R., Rook, G., Swana, G. T. *et al.* (1981). Autoantibodies to cartilage and type II collagen in relapsing polychondritis and other rheumatic disease. *Ann. Rheum. Dis.*, **40**, 473–9
69. Rajapakse, D. A. and Bywaters, E. G. L. (1974). Cell-mediated immunity to cartilage proteoglycan in relapsing polychondritis. *Clin. Exp. Immunol.*, **16**, 497–502
70. Conti, J. A., Coliccho, M. D. and Havard, L. M. (1988). Thymoma, myasthenia gravis and relapsing polychondritis. *Ann. Intern. Med.*, **109** (2), 163–4

71. Pope, R. M., Ludgate, M. E. and McGregor, A. M. (1986). Observations on Graves' ophthalmopathy; pathology and pathogenesis. In McGregor, A. M. (ed.) *Immunology of Endocrine Diseases*, pp. 161–80. (Lancaster: MTP)
72. Weetman, A. P. (1986). HLA-DR antigen expression and autoimmunity. In McGregor, A. M. (ed.) *Immunology of Endocrine Diseases*, pp. 143–59. (Lancaster: MTP)
73. Arnold, I., Levison, B., Zweiman, B. and Lisak, R. P. (1987). Immunopathogenesis and treatment of myasthenia gravis. *J. Clin. Immunol.*, **7** (3), 187
74. Lefvert, A. K. (1986). Auto-anti-idiotypic immunity and acetylcholine receptors. *Concepts Immunopathol.*, **3**, 285–310

Index